EVERY DAY A MIRACLE

SUCCESS STORIES WITH SOUND THERAPY

EVERY DAY A MIRACLE

SUCCESS STORIES WITH SOUND THERAPY

BY DORINNE S. DAVIS, MA, CCC-A, FAAA, RCTC, BARA

KALCO PUBLISHING, LLC

Supervising Editor: Ruth Cruz
Director of Operations: Eric S. Kalugin
Cover & Layout Design: Ruth Cruz
Cover Art: Ricardo Martínez

Kalco Publishing, LLC.
Landing, New Jersey

Kalco Publishing, LLC.
51 King Road
Landing, NJ 07850

For information or to order:
Tel: 973.347.3509
Fax: 973.601.9334
info@kalcopublishing.com

Library of Congress Control Number: 2005930251

Davis, Dorinne S.
  Every Day A Miracle: Success Stories with Sound Therapy
  ISBN: 978-0-9622326-4-0 (pbk.)

1. Success stories with sound-based therapies using the application of the DETP™ at The Davis Center, sound-based therapies, sound therapy, therapeutic programs

2. Health, well-being, alternative therapy
3. Auditory Integration Training, Tomatis, BioAcoustics
4. Autism, ADD, ADHD, PDD, PDD-NOS, dyslexia, Williams syndrome, Tourette's syndrome, CAPD, Central Auditory Processing Disorder

Printed in the United States of America

10 9 8 7 6 5 4 3 2 1

DEDICATIONS

My heartfelt thanks are extended to all of the individuals and families who shared their personal sagas so that the world will hear of their successes.

I would also like to say thank you to *The Davis Center* staff for supporting these clients and thousands more that visit our center while making the exceptional changes that we see everyday, our "miracles".

I wish to say a special thank you to Michael Allen for his help in obtaining all of the stories, to my husband Eric, for his editing support, and to Ruth Cruz for the beautiful cover and the finishing touches.

Finally, I thank my family for always supporting and encouraging me to explore new concepts, and taking the leaps forward with me.

Dorinne

CONTENTS

PREFACE

Each day at *The Davis Center*, someone shares an "AHA!" moment. Every day someone on the staff will ask, "What's the miracle of the day?" and it's because *Every Day A Miracle* takes place at *The Davis Center*. On the day I received my first copy of *Sound Bodies through Sound Therapy*, I knew I had to share our "wow" moments with others. The best way to do this would be directly from the clients or parents of the clients themselves.

The reason *The Davis Center* has these success stories to share is because of how our clients fit into *The Tree of Sound Enhancement Therapy™*. Clients receive therapies in the correct order for maximum success and get retested periodically to make sure the program continues to be appropriate. I developed the *Diagnostic Evaluation for Therapy Protocol* (*DETP™*) which determines the correct progression for the therapies to follow. As long as the progression is followed, success is possible. *The Tree* represents the voice-ear-brain connection in its totality.

For those who haven't read *Sound Bodies through Sound Therapy*, *The Tree of Sound Enhancement Therapy* represents the connections between the various sound-based therapies available today. *The Tree* evolved as I became trained, certified, and worked with all of the major sound-based therapies. I saw connections and differences between the various therapies. With my experience as an audiologist, educator/teacher, and my research over the years, I was able to figure out these connections and differences. I brought together the concepts of the anatomy and physiology of the ear and body, early childhood development skills, how a child learns academically, audiological testing, and vibrational sound. Interestingly, it was the impact of sound and vibration on the body that has been the most important.

Although historical greats like Pythagoras taught us that music could heal, it wasn't until Dr. Alfred Tomatis discovered the connection between the voice, the ear, and the brain in the 1950's that the concept of physiological change occurring with sound or music stimulation became better understood. Dr. Tomatis' concepts were first confirmed at the French Academy of Science in 1957 and again in 1960. His concepts became known as "The Tomatis Effect". Forty-seven years later my research has extended these concepts. My research was presented in 2004 at the International Association of Logopedics and Phoniatrics in Brisbane, Australia, and at the Acoustical Society of America in San Diego, CA and is now known as *The Davis Addendum™ to the Tomatis Effect*. The combination of "The Tomatis Effect" and *The Davis Addendum to the Tomatis Effect* make up *The Tree of Sound Enhancement Therapy*. It is this *Cycle of Sound™*, created by the impact of sound vibration in the voice-ear-brain connection that makes *The Tree* concept work.

Once *The Tree of Sound Enhancement Therapy* hierarchy was in place, it was only logical to find a way to identify where on *The Tree* clients would best be helped by sound therapy. While writing *Sound Bodies through Sound Therapy*, I knew that I had to find a way to accomplish this. The *Diagnostic Evaluation for Therapy Protocol* was created as a test battery to provide evaluative results at every level of *The Tree*. A starting place is identified as well as a suggested series of therapies that will help the person begin to make positive change.

This book, *Every Day A Miracle: Success Stories with Sound Therapy* is a sharing of personal stories of people who have used the *DETP* as the entry point for services. It is important because it demonstrates that some people need more than one therapy to achieve the desired change. Without the proper starting point and order, some parents have reported that their children are not maintaining the changes received by only one therapy. Others report that their child had a negative response; or that the child did well but something seemed to be missing. Before the therapy protocol begins, the person receiving therapy or the parents of the child receiving therapy need to understand that more than one therapy may be needed to get to "the miracle". Sometimes the miracles are not seen until all the proper foundational changes are in place with the baseline therapies. It may seem like nothing happened with some of the baseline therapies to the beholder, but since sound impacts the body on a cellular level, changes are constantly taking place. To achieve the leaps and bounds, as reported in this book, all baseline therapies had to be in place. All of the clients mentioned in this book used the *DETP* for guidance in the administration of sound-based therapies.

I have asked my clients and their families to share their experiences with others. What you are about to read are 16 personal stories— these stories reveal their lives before, during, and after their experiences with sound therapies. Some of the stories are still in progress, as the individual may not be finished with their sound therapy protocol provided by the DETP. Others have achieved their goals and the outcome of positive changes remains. All have a wonderful story to tell.

The beginning of each chapter's story quotes "the miracle" found in each story. Each personal story shares a little about their life, what the person was like prior to coming to *The Davis Center* and takes you through the steps of their sound therapy journey. After each story, I have added brief comments to clarify a few points. The stories always leave me with a warm and fuzzy feeling. I hope you will feel the same.

CHAPTER ONE

Matthew   Autism

"He's responding more like a normal child,
it's almost instantaneous."

Blue Hill, Maine: Cynthia gets comfortable on her couch as she takes a deep breath and prepares to tell her story.

*M*atthew was developing well as a young child. He was very alert and could pick his head up at birth. He crawled early and even began walking early. But at the age of two, Matthew started demonstrating some unusual changes. He was not responding to questions or instructions. I would have to repeat myself two or three times. There are times when I could see the wheels turning in his head, but it would take a few seconds to process the question or the instruction. Sometimes the response would take up to five minutes.

For some reason, Matthew would respond well to the alarm on the microwave. When the alarm would go off, he would look straight at it. I thought he responded to the microwave because he was hungry. He also responded better to his older sister Michelle. Maybe because they were closer together in age or maybe he just formed a special bond with her, I'm not really sure. It's hard to diagnose your own child. The signs you see can lead you to conclusions that may not be true. So while I was thinking that he had picked up some behavioral issues, the healthcare officials at the local hospital thought Matthew might have some level of hearing loss. Because Matthew was non-responsive, they believed he was going deaf.

Even though he had been a fast developer, his development started to slow down. He had enough language to say things he wanted like "apple." But talking was too bothersome for him. It seemed that he didn't want a great deal to do with language at all. He didn't like to construct complete sentences.

My husband Dwayne and I took Matthew to see his pediatrician, Dr. Baroody. He suggested that my husband attend a Defeat Autism Now or DAN conference, and gather all the literature he could. I didn't really have a good grasp of what exactly autism was. When I learned that autism dealt with impaired communication and social skills, I knew that Matthew was going to need specialized attention. The DAN conference had plenty of booths outside the lecture hall where different companies, pharmaceuticals and informational centers were setup. *The Davis Center* had a booth there as well. Dr. Baroody happened to recognize a doctor's name in the literature and told us that Dr. Bock and he had been lab partners at one time. So at Dr. Baroody's suggestion, we started taking Matthew to see Dr. Bock. Matthew was seven years old at the time.

Dr. Bock was a medical doctor. He took blood tests and found Matthew to have a leaky gut. He prescribed supplements and different IVs, among them were magnesium and glutathione. Dr. Bock wasn't specifically addressing Matthew's autism. However Dr. Bock had worked with Dorinne Davis in conferences and knew very well of her work and her successes with autistic children. Dr. Bock referred Matthew to *The Davis Center* in 2003 when Matthew was eleven years old.

Based on Dorinne's recommendations we'd have to travel to New Jersey and stay for what could be fifteen days at a time. This was not going to be an easy task, but we managed. Dwayne would drive down with us and then fly back to Maine. Sometimes my daughter, Michelle, would have to stay with her grandparents, but we would bring her with us as often as we could. Sometimes she would drive down with us and fly back with Dwayne. It was hard, because we seldom separate as a family. If we would have to split up we've always tried to make up for it in other ways and do special things together. Michelle has had to make some major adjustments in her life, but she has been a great support to her brother. We never in our wildest dreams would have chosen to place Michelle in this situation. She has understood that we've had to do this and has always been very supportive of our decisions.

When we went to New Jersey, we usually stayed at a hotel. I have a sister in Pennsylvania and we tried to stay there as often as we could when we went down, but more often than not, my sister would have to come visit us at our hotel.

I really had no expectations of *The Davis Center* at all. I wasn't sure what was going to happen when we got there the first time. I originally thought that Dorinne was going to do the AIT and then we would go home. I was shocked when they did the first test and Dorinne told me that I should follow AIT immediately with the Tomatis® program. Dorinne explained that each diagnosis is specialized to the individual. The *Diagnostic Evaluation for Therapy Protocol* is a careful evaluation process where Dorinne decides the right time to start each therapy. There is perfect timing for everything, but there is also a wrong time to start a therapy. In Matthew's case, it would benefit him greatly if they had him start with AIT and follow this immediately with the first session of Tomatis.

Dorinne explained her findings further. Matthew had issues with the muscles in his ears. They weren't doing what they should. I was astounded to learn that certain behaviors he displayed were connected with his hearing. These connections had never been made before. He would chew on things. He would push on his chin. Dorinne explained that he was trying to stimulate the muscles in his ear himself. He had other behaviors and they all seemed to be connected with Matthew's ability to hear. I decided that Dorinne knew what she was talking about and I was ready to see if she could help Matthew.

Matthew began the ten days of AIT and directly after, he started Tomatis. He was to do two 15-day sessions with thirty days in between. Then we did two 8-day boosts. Some of Matthew's old behaviors began to come back during Tomatis. Matthew started pulling on his collar and the sleeves of his shirt. Dorinne was quick to explain that some muscles are understimulated and some are overstimulated. Dorinne mentioned that she had seen a case where one girl's shirt sleeves bothered her and she couldn't stand a collar around her neck. Matthew was experiencing the same thing. These sound-based therapies cause stimulation. Hearing is a key note to many different things, and hearing is connected to the body in more ways than we can begin to understand.

Matthew was exhausted from the therapy. It can make them tired. The listening does so much to the body that it just wears them down. Sometimes he would fall asleep during sessions; he would fall asleep as soon as we got back to the hotel room.

During Christmas vacation, we were able to do therapy at home. Matthew did The Listening Program®, which is Mozart filtered music with certain nature sounds. For thirty minutes, Matthew would listen through a set of headphones to these specially arranged CD's. He has also used the LiFT (Listening Fitness Training) program. Each time he listens, it has become easier and easier for Matthew to read. He had weekly reading assignments like the *Twelve Days of Christmas*. He would read into a microphone and he could hear himself while Mozart played in the background. Then the music segment would change to play Gregorian chants without the microphone. In these segments, the filters and the balance settings were changed. The balance settings were changed because Matthew needed his right ear stimulated more. The right sends sound to the left side of the brain and it is the left side of the brain that processes language. Communication enters the right ear and travels around the head to finally be processed on the left side. Now it made sense to me why it took him so long to respond to questions or instructions.

The most astounding thing we noticed about Matthew happened during AIT. When spoken to he immediately "got it". He has continued to get better and better at processing information and responding to questions and instructions. He still hesitates sometimes, but he is getting better. He's responding more like a normal child, it's almost instantaneous.

Matthew has a more spontaneous use of language. He uses sentences now when he communicates. He is more focused on the world around him and he is a much calmer person than he used to be. When he returned to school, the teachers were very surprised. Dorinne stressed that if the child can be put through therapy before puberty, the process is better. The teachers learned this first hand. Before sound therapy teachers worked with him so cautiously, just trying to find any way for him to survive on a day to day basis in school. But now we are looking for ways to get him more advanced.

STORY RESPONSE

Matthew was 11-years old when I first met him. You could tell he was going to be a tall boy from his gangly physique and sure enough, he has continued to grow each time we see him. At his last visit, Matthew was 13½-years old and about 5 foot 6 inches and still growing.

Matthew was referred to me from a Defeat Autism Now (DAN) practitioner, Dr. Bock. *The Davis Center* has been working closely with DAN practitioners and other alternative practice physicians with good results. We admit that our sound therapies are not the be all and end all for all people. However, I do believe that we are the starting place. Sound therapy enhancing stimulation prepares the body for maximum sensory reception. We have demonstrated that other services like occupational, speech, physical, and other therapies have a better chance to build on the sensory foundation established, achieving faster and more in depth results for those complementary therapies. For example, many children who have had speech services for ten years with no significant change, have been able to eliminate speech therapy, approximately two months after the basic Tomatis method program had corrected their issues.

When parents have to travel long distances for our services, which so many do, my goal is to get the person to a level where most of the therapies can be done with home programs. Once Matthew was ready, I was able to introduce some of the home-based therapies. These typically focus on the upper *Trunk* or lower *Leaves and Branches* segments of my analogy of *The Tree*.

Matthew's mother reported that his reading improved each time he used the LiFT program at home. One of the final pieces of the voice-ear-brain connection is the ability to use one's own voice for personal body maintenance. Once Matthew became more comfortable with hearing his own voice, he was better able to use this new response for supporting the positive changes he experienced. This was especially true with regard to his reading skills. He was better able to listen and process the sounds as he read them, thereby helping him to better process the language he was reading.

The definitions of "hearing" versus "listening" are important. Many people believe them to be the same, including Matthew's mother at the time. *The Davis Center* intake includes many different tests, one is a hearing test and another is a listening test. When I test hearing, I typically test for hypersensitive hearing. What I am testing for is the minimum level that our ear hears sound 50% of the time. This is called "threshold". I test at many frequencies. This test should not be considered a complete audiological assessment. I actually include more frequencies than the standard protocol and look at different parameters of the hearing function. I also test for listening. The "Listening Test" measures when a person begins to tune into sound. It requires a person to mentally be aware of the presence of a sound. It should not be considered similar to a hearing test. These test responses and the interpretation of the Listening Test are evaluated differently from a hearing test. Most people have better hearing than listening skills.

When I address specific issues with my sound-based therapy protocol, I typically address hearing issues before listening issues. In Matthew's case, for hearing purposes, I needed to work on retraining how one muscle in his middle ear worked before addressing how the entire ear used sound stimulation. Listening requires the use of sound stimulation. Hearing and listening are addressed by two different types of sound-based therapies. Hearing is represented by the *Root System* of *The Tree* analogy, while listening is represented by the *Trunk System*. The therapies also affect change in different ways and at different levels, so the body's responses are often different.

By emphasizing both hearing and listening for Matthew, he was able to move forward with good, consistent, positive progress. It's exciting to meet Matthew when he comes to *The Davis Center* because now he can look you in the eye and respond appropriately. He is learning at a faster pace and enjoys his new sense of awareness and responsiveness.

CHAPTER TWO

Mary

Neurodevelopmental Issues
Chromosome Imbalance

> "That floored me because that was
> her first sentence, at the age of five."

Indianapolis, Indiana: Nancy looks concerned as she begins to form her thoughts. Then she relaxes and shares her memories.

*M*ary was a difficult pregnancy. She stopped growing in utero and was delivered around 34-weeks gestation. When she was born, it was difficult to get her to start breathing. She has an abnormality in one of her chromosomes, the third chromosome in fact. Throughout her infancy, she didn't eat right. The doctors gave me reason for concern when they suggested a generic diagnosis. All they simply said was that her development would be delayed. Obviously, we felt that we needed to know a little bit more than that.

Every development skill was delayed. Mary didn't walk until she was 2-years old. She was five with no vocabulary. "Dadda" and "Momma" was all she knew. We used a little bit of sign language because her speech was so incomprehensible. It was like she had her own language. We started to understand it, but no one else could get it at all. She was also very sensitive to loud noises and crowds, as she would get hyper. When we entered a large crowd, or loud music was playing, she would start screaming and crying.

When she was 4½-years old, we got tickets to see *Disney on Ice** at the Conseco Fieldhouse. She loved Disney and absolutely loved Mickey, but when the crowd started cheering and the lights came on, she was not happy. She started putting her hands over

---

* *Disney on Ice* is owned/operated by Disney Enterprises, Inc./Pixar Animation Studios.

her ears. We tried moving around the arena and seeing if there was anyway she could enjoy the show. We ended up leaving before it really even got started. That wasn't all. The fourth of July always sent her into a crazy fit and fire trucks would set her off shaking, screaming and crying hysterically.

Because of her delay in language development, she attended speech therapy for two years. It was an iffy situation on a daily basis. If she was happy she would play, but when one thing went wrong, she would cry. She was very emotional. The slightest thing could make her change her mood in a heartbeat from being happy to suddenly crying. Not knowing what to do, we tried many things. Through the early intervention program in the public school system, we tried physical therapy, occupational therapy, and speech therapy. The speech therapist recommended a center in Detroit, Michigan. The director evaluated Mary and asked her questions basically just to get her to talk. Then the director and I talked about it. She told me that they could help her there eventually, but Mary was too up and down emotionally to really do that much with her at the time. Mary just didn't have the attention span to be able to effectively work with her. So the director recommended coming back to Detroit when Mary's attention span was better. She totally left us in the dark.

We returned home with little idea about what to do except ask our pediatrician and speech therapist for help. They had a few recommendations for how to get Mary's attention span under control. They wanted us to put Mary on Prozac®† and Focalin™‡. Then they took her off Prozac and put her on Zoloft®§. They took

---

† Prozac® is a registered trademark of Eli Lilly and Company.

‡ Focalin™ is manufactured and distributed by Novartis Pharmaceuticals Corporation.

§ Zoloft® is manufactured and distributed by Pfizer Inc.

her off Zoloft and put her on Seroquel®**, which helped her language increase. She started using more words, but her attention span wasn't there yet. Then the doctor put her on Straterra®†† along with the Seroquel. She only lasted two weeks. They said that Straterra will take awhile to see if it works, but you know right away if it's not going to work. Mary gained a temper from it. It was around this time that I heard about Tomatis.

We heard about Tomatis through a friend of my brother who had a son with autism. He was taking his son to a Tomatis center. I was definitely sold on Tomatis because his son was diagnosed when he was four and by the time he was twelve, he was functioning as a normal twelve year old. So, I got on the Internet and started looking for this Tomatis center. When I looked up Tomatis, I found out that only five places in the United States offered Tomatis. Being from Indiana, *The Davis Center* stood out because it was closer than any other one.

Speaking with Dorinne, it seemed like Tomatis was something we had to try for Mary. But when we actually met with Dorinne, I learned more about the process. The initial assessment was very thorough. During the *Diagnostic Evaluation for Therapy Protocol* or *DETP*, they had us fill out a questionnaire and she went over everything with us. During the initial assessment, Mary wouldn't do it by herself. She had to sit on my lap during the first hearing test. But she did well otherwise. They put us in a booth and Mary had to wear headphones. Dorinne asked her questions and Mary stayed focused the entire time. She really listened to Dorinne. It just all seemed very thorough the way Mary responded to the

---

** Seroquel® is manufactured and distributed by AstraZeneca Pharmaceuticals LP.
†† Straterra® is manufactured and distributed by Eli Lilly and Company.

questions and the way Dorinne read her body responses. Then Dorinne explained her findings and she really seemed to know her stuff. Everything sounded logical and I knew it was worth trying.

The thing was that we weren't going to be doing Tomatis first. That's what I thought we were going to be doing. Dorinne explained that there is a right time for each therapy. The first thing Dorinne suggested was Auditory Integration Training which lasted two weeks. At first, it was hard to get Mary to remain quiet and sit still. She wouldn't wear the headphones either. We would do sessions twice a day with a 4-hour break in between. By the fourth session, Mary walked in and put the headphones on herself. It was really great.

At the end of AIT, we took five days off and then went straight into Tomatis. Mary really took to it. She never tried to take her headphones off like the other kids. She actually had fun playing with other kids. She was having fun with everything about it.

Language development was one thing we noticed right away. When we were taking her to *The Davis Center*, I brought her to the first two days and my husband brought her the next two days. When it was my turn to take her again on the fifth day she asked, "Daddy go me again." That floored me because that was her first sentence, at the age of five.

We have since had two more 15-day sessions. The third session was split between an 8-day and a 7-day session. We had a two month break between those two sessions, and then we did two more 8-day sessions after that, and had a four month break between those.

Mary is still a little hyper, and sometimes she has a problem sitting still. But her sensitivity to loud noises has changed. She doesn't scream and cry to loud noises anymore. Driving home one day, a police car drove by with the blaring sirens and Mary pointed at it with awe. In the past it had been the kind of thing to throw her into a crazy fit. I was stunned.

I can't say enough about her language development. She is talking so much clearer than she ever talked before. The last time we went to *The Davis Center* was in August. She had made tremendous strides. She started asking for something to drink by saying, "Water, please." She initiated connections by saying things like "Hugs." I melted the first time she said, "I love you Mommy." Her younger brother Charlie got a nickname. Mary started calling him Char for short. She was getting more comfortable with language and starting to master it herself.

When we go to *The Davis Center*, we stay with my mother and father because they live nearby. The first time we stayed with them was the first time Mary had been away from her father for a month. It was hard for us to work out the details and juggle everything. I know it was harder on Mary being away from her father for that long. Mary has adjusted, and now when we go to my parent's for anything, even for just Christmas, Mary asks, "Am I going listening?" She looks forward to it.

STORY RESPONSE

Mary is an adorable little girl. When I first met her, she was 4½-years old. She was all over the place. Mary's limited speech was very difficult to understand and her mother had to interpret for her. It was obvious that Mary wanted to carry on a conversation in the worst way. She would use single words interspersed between strings of gibberish that sounded like sentence structure. Mary was also extremely hypersensitive to sound.

My *DETP* is able to identify three different types of hearing hypersensitivities, as they pertain to my analogy of *The Tree of Sound Enhancement Therapy*. My initial *DETP* typically consists of either a partial or full battery of tests. The partial is for children who do not have sufficient language skills for me to obtain information about the *Leaves and Branches* skill level of *The Tree* analogy. These children typically are very sensitive to touch at the ear canal, so one type of hearing hypersensitivity test is not included in the partial *DETP*. Mary's *DETP* only tested for two types of hearing hypersensitivity and both types were present.

Even though her parents initially thought that Mary would benefit from the Tomatis method, Mary needed to start with Bérard's Auditory Integration Training. This in order to address one type of hearing hypersensitivity that showed up on her hearing sensitivity threshold test. Depending upon the interpretation of the test data, when this type of hearing hypersensitivity shows up, one typically needs to start therapy with Auditory Integration Training. AIT establishes the proper foundation for muscle response in the middle ear for the transmission of sound to the inner ear and subsequently to the brain.

It makes sense that if sound is painful to listen to, the person will react. Typically there are three types of responses. First the person overreacts, covers their ears, runs around wildly, cries, screams, throws tantrums, or needs to leave the room; secondly the person shuts down by turning off the sound at the brain and therefore doesn't tune into what is necessary or important; or thirdly the person responds inwardly, retreating into their own little world and only responding externally when drawn out of their inner world. Once sound is more comfortable, the person can then begin to listen to what is happening around them. Mary is now more comfortable with sound and can enjoy the world around her. She can tune into what is being said by others and can learn the various parts of language.

Dr. Tomatis' laws can be summarized as "The voice can only produce what the ear hears." For Mary, her speech is becoming clearer and more easily understood because of her ability to hear the sounds of speech more clearly. Along the way, we have worked on developing her listening skills. Listening is a key component to furthering the development of her language skills. The Tomatis method works on listening skills. Listening is a more advanced skill set than the hearing function. Hearing is the body's response to the transmission of sound to the brain. Listening involves a mental process, and is therefore a higher functioning skill set. Because of this, in Mary's case the Tomatis method was not the place to start her therapy protocol.

Mary was able to accept her headphones because she sensed that changes were being made and felt comfortable. Mary's mother reported that Mary looked forward to coming for the therapies, demonstrating that Mary knew she felt good about herself and that she had responded to the therapies. Mary liked her "new me" and she wanted more.

The suggested *DETP* therapy order for Mary to receive therapies was to start with Auditory Integration Training first, and then proceed to the Tomatis method. It was also suggested that she start BioAcoustics® after the second session of Tomatis. BioAcoustics has proven to be one of the most important components of the voice-ear-brain connection because BioAcoustics works at the cellular level when making change. Often these changes are not immediately an "AHA!" moment, yet they can be. However, incorporating BioAcoustics when indicated can be the missing supportive factor for our clients in making even greater change for the long run. Before determining any advanced levels of sound therapies to address the *Leaves and Branches* of *The Tree,* Mary will further benefit from the support of BioAcoustics. BioAcoustics supports the long term results.

CHAPTER THREE

Candy

Learning Issues, Adoption
Sensory Integration Disorder

> "She could start feeling pain. When she fell and
> scraped her knee, she was crying real tears."

Philadelphia, Pennsylvania: Donna considers her thoughts with a smile on her face as she recalls the past few years with her daughter. She also remembers some memories that were rather upsetting at the time.

*C*andy was adopted from Guatemala. We got her at 4½-months. When we got her, she was sick with something commonly referred to as chronic bronchitis. She would cough all night long. I had to sleep with her sitting up in a chair. The doctor at the local clinic told us that it came from chronic sinus trouble. Like tonsils, adenoids can become enlarged and block the breathing. Candy had her adenoids removed when she was two years old. Even after the operation she was still continuously sick and continued to cough all night. I should have seen the signs. I knew something wasn't right. The professionals we were taking her to weren't spotting any other problems. They ran plenty of tests on her, but they just kept treating Candy for chronic bronchitis. Our family doctor told us there was no such thing. He suggested taking her to the children's hospital where they insisted on putting tubes in her ears. They tested her hearing and said that it was fine, but enlarged adenoids can sometimes cause ear infections. The tubes helped ventilate the ear and drain the fluids that could gather there.

We never once made a connection between her behavior and her sickness. Being quiet and starting to talk late were being attributed to the complications doctors had found with her adenoids and ultimately her ears. Her other behaviors weren't symptomatic of her medical complications. She was a very difficult child, and our life was a bit stressful. I knew something wasn't right, but I couldn't call it. I could not take Candy to the mall or to work. She would spin in circles or run and hide between clothes. When we were out, it seemed like she was unmanageable; but it wasn't like that at home, only when we went some place.

However, she had some behaviors at home too. She hated whenever someone would try to read to her, and would throw a fit. She wanted everything loud. She liked the music left on at night and always wanted the volume turned up a bit too much. Candy didn't look people in the eye when they talked to her. She also didn't cry much. She was always putting herself into dangerous situations. She would climb trees or the monkey bars and hang upside down off of them. But if she hurt herself and was bleeding, she wouldn't cry. Although when she was an infant, I needed to hold her tight and jump up and down to get her to stop crying. It never occurred to me that these behaviors were all connected. Loud music, not looking people in the eye, not feeling pain and not crying don't seem to connect at all.

Candy had this other thing too. Candy hated to walk across the bathroom floor. She hated the coldness on her feet. She would make a path with towels. Then one night, I was watching a primetime show on sensory integration disorder and the show talked about many of the things that Candy was doing. These were the things that didn't add together. While the show was offering me a way of dealing with Candy, I was tuned into the idea that maybe Candy had this sensory integration disorder. I started looking up sensory integration disorder everywhere I found a resource. I found *The Out of Sync Child* by Carol Kranowitz. The book outlines a few strategies and also mentions Tomatis. I still hadn't made the connection yet. I went into the school and asked for them to test Candy for sensory integration disorder. They looked at me as if I had three heads. Just to appease me, they did try testing her, but it took all year and in the long run amounted to nothing.

Taking it all in and trying to come up with solutions on my own, I was coming to the conclusion that Candy's problems were with her sight and being visually overstimulated. Liking loud music aside, her problems seemed to be with her sight because I thought it had something to do with light. She was addicted to the television. I had to pry her away and she would throw a temper tantrum. The television changed her behavior drastically. It literally altered her behavior. I also thought her problem was visual because of what happened when I got her this particular jigsaw puzzle for Christmas. It was heavily patterned and it even made me feel overstimulated. Candy kept pushing pieces on the floor and then she would hang upside down to pick up the pieces. After learning what that was about, I was able to see that Candy did that to realign her brain. I also noticed her doing that when her homework became too much for her. She would push a pencil on the floor.

Being overstimulated, she would hang herself upside down on the monkey bars and on tree branches. This was why she was always putting herself in danger. Another thing she needed to do was bounce or spin. I remembered this from when she was an infant and she would cry. Even though she had since quit crying, she still wanted that stimulation of when I would jump up and down to get her to quit crying. So we got her a Sit-and-Spin. When she watched too much television, we would put her on the Sit-and-Spin to get her back. By "get her back" I mean that when she was watching television, she would be mesmerized or almost like hypnotized. We would have to get her away from the television. She threw unbelievable fits when we had to turn the television off to go anywhere. But even when we didn't have to go anywhere, we knew she should only have so much television. So we would actually have to wrestle with her and get her on the Sit-and-Spin. At first she would throw a fit, but she would feel better right away. One day, it dawned on me how special it was that Candy had learned her own strategy to realign the brain.

She had taught herself other coping strategies as well. I mean, to paint an entire picture of Candy, she was quiet in school. Teachers often remarked that Candy was so quiet they didn't even know she was there. She didn't bother anyone. She pretty much kept to herself. But sometimes the teachers misinterpreted her inactivity. Candy was only trying to cope with things in her own way. When she was getting bullied by a student to buy items that were written on a list, Candy showed me the list so that I could purchase the items. I told her that we weren't going to handle it that way. I was going to show the list to her teacher. When I took the list into the school to show her teachers, they told me that Candy had asked for another list. Her teachers saw Candy as being as much at fault because she was actually asking for a list. They wouldn't acknowledge that Candy might have been afraid or could see no other way out of the situation. I could see it as a coping strategy, but they couldn't see the big picture. It was my feeling all along that some people just didn't get it, not just with my child and definitely not with children like mine. I don't know how to say it any better than they just didn't get it.

In kindergarten, Candy could not learn her alphabet. At the end of first grade, the school routinely conducted a psychological education evaluation and they brought it to my attention that

Candy had auditory processing issues. The psychologist of the school sent us to an audiologist. We were sent to an audiologist in the suburbs of Philadelphia, but she only did the Fast ForWord® program. Fast ForWord is a sound-based therapy that uses interactive, computer-based training programs for people with language-learning difficulties. The audiologist sent us to an institute where they do occupational therapy for children with sensory integration disorders.

Through all of these various resources, I was learning more about what was going on with my daughter, but nothing had really fallen into place yet. I was still trying to seek help in the schools with Candy's teachers, but they just weren't getting it that my daughter had issues that needed to be addressed. They would just look at me like I was crazy or it was a waste of time to pursue. They were looking at it as if sensory integration was only experimental. Their solutions were to just put the kids on Ritalin. I was moving my daughter around a little from school to school trying to find one that would really work for her. Two different schools told me to put my child on Ritalin®*. From the second and third grade, Candy was in a school for children who learn differently. My feeling was that they didn't seem to "get it" either. My frustration was that parents thought they had found a place to take their kids and give them a place to learn. But even this school that claimed to be geared specifically for helping my child didn't get it. If I asked them for anything special that could benefit Candy, they didn't have it. The teachers were looking at all the kids they had and teaching them as a whole rather than individually.

It was recommended to me to put Candy through counseling. Candy was not able to express her emotions, and her

---

* Ritalin® is manufactured and distributed by Novartis Pharmaceuticals Corporation.

reactions to things were misread. When I tried to show the teachers information about sensory integration disorders, they would look at the information and just ignore it. They weren't listening to me. If it wasn't taught to them from another professional, they didn't think it beneficial. They definitely wouldn't let a parent introduce them to new things.

Obviously, Candy needed something else. She needed something that would actually work for her. Every way I turned, I was becoming more and more frustrated. When I tried to get her a little extra tutoring help, the teachers would ask if she was really a special needs student or if I just wanted extra help for her. They came to the conclusion that I just wanted it for her and she didn't really need any specialized treatment in school. But I knew Candy had some issues that weren't on the surface. She was my daughter. I noticed. People who didn't know her wouldn't notice those issues.

The Occupational Therapist working with Candy referred us to Dorinne Davis and recommended the Lindamood-Bell® program, a multisensory awareness program that helps students develop sensory-cognitive functions as well as basic reading skills. So I made arrangements and had Dorinne evaluate Candy with the *Diagnostic Evaluation for Therapy Protocol*. After evaluating Candy, Dorinne sat down with me and explained some things that really made sense. The *DETP* reflects Dorinne's analogy of *The Tree*. Dorinne explained that the initial hearing sensitivity test indicated some things about Candy's hearing status. Dorinne explained everything to me. Now learning about the details of the middle ear, everything I had experienced with Candy fell into place. The tubes in Candy's ears and her enlarged adenoids all had something to do with her middle ear. But more phenomenal than that was how it explained all of Candy's behaviors.

I thought to myself that this was the missing piece. *The Davis Center* was the missing piece of Candy's puzzle. *The Davis Center* was going to find the solution to the puzzle. The little quirky things about Candy were starting to make sense. Her need for loud music, but being quiet in school and her behavior around noises in public had all seemed so strange. The pieces didn't quite add up before, but they were starting to now. When she wouldn't cry when she would hurt herself, it was because of the connection between her sense of hearing and the skin that she couldn't feel pain. That's why she would put herself in dangerous situations. She also wouldn't look anyone in the eye when they were talking to her. She would always look off one way or another. She looked like she wasn't paying attention. In fact she just didn't know from what direction the sounds were coming. The answers I needed and desperately searched for all along were finally here.

The pediatricians and Ear, Nose, and Throat or ENT doctors would test her and say that her hearing was fine. Actually there were certain frequencies she couldn't hear well, while there were things she could hear that no one else could. I was starting to see it all fit together now. She liked loud music because she could hardly hear it, but she couldn't stand crowded public places because she could hear that all too well.

I had noticed that if I talked quietly to her, I got a better response from her. Yelling at her got me nowhere. As I was learning more about her hearing issues, I remembered a teacher who was soft spoken and talked very quietly. Candy did well in her class. I had never made that connection before. Dorinne had made so much sense of it all.

I saw change on the first day of her Auditory Integration Training. After our first half hour session, I remember saying something to Candy. She looked me in the eye that day and it made me cry. She was also quite calm and more compliant. Before all this, Candy couldn't tell us how she felt. From the first day of AIT, conversations started to increase. She wanted to try new foods, and she was definitely more agreeable.

Candy's perception of the environment around her was also changing. She didn't know where she was in the world. The air on her skin felt different. She needed something on her arms and feet. We cut out the feet on knee-high socks to put on her arms. She had to readjust with walking too. The changes that were taking place were taking place with everything about her. When she fell and scraped her knee, she cried real tears. We knew that she started feeling pain, and she was more real to us than ever. Her laughter and her tears were more real. Her emotions were more real.

We did AIT for two weeks and it was like I had a new kid. We went straight into Tomatis the next week. But there was something different this time. Candy regressed. She wanted to be wrapped in a blanket and held like a baby. Tomatis took my 8-year old back to needing to be treated like a baby. Dorinne explained that the sense of hearing affects every part of your body. Candy needed to adjust. Nurture the moment and let it go. Candy started sucking her thumb. It was like she was helpless. I wanted my AIT kid back.

Dorinne ended up taking Candy slower through Tomatis. We had done two 15-day sessions with a three- to four-week break in between. Positive changes occurred throughout Tomatis as well. Our bonding became stronger. Candy's love and acceptance of me was stronger and it came from a different place. It came from her heart and not her head.

We've been doing an 8-day boost every three months and

we've done three so far. The one thing I started to worry about was that her school environment could cause her to regress. The teachers at her school saw the differences after Candy went through AIT and Tomatis. But they didn't support the program. I decided to keep Candy in the Lindamood-Bell program. We have also participated in Dorinne's *Read-Spell-Comprehend*® program, which incorporates some of the Lindamood-Bell programs with an auditory and developmental twist. But we went back to the Lindamood-Bell program because it is closer. We take the train half an hour to the Lindamood-Bell learning center right here in Philadelphia. It's like getting tutored one-on-one all week long. It's a 12-week program. If kids don't get it in the twelve weeks, they have to go longer.

At the time, I am looking for a closer school I can send Candy to that is perfect for her. Some schools offer the Fast ForWord program, but they are not doing it the right way. The teachers aren't really doing it when the kids don't want to participate. A teacher might ask, "Do you want to do Fast ForWord today or work on your parts in the play?" Of course, the kids don't benefit from it if it isn't being done consistently. I have found a new school that seems like it is going to be a decent school for Candy. It has Occupational Therapists on staff and it seems like the whole school gets it. They understand what is going on with these kids and they have the resources available to work with them.

My other daughter, Mary, has also benefited from what *The Davis Center* can do. She is an "A" student. I did therapy with Mary because she does not test well. I was originally just going to have Mary tutored for her SAT and put her through the Lindamood-Bell program. But from what I learned with Candy, I thought maybe it's not a reading comprehension problem. I thought maybe it could be her hearing. So we tested her at *The Davis Center* and she did have some sound sensitivities. She does feel better. One day, she told Dorinne, "I can't explain it, I just feel better." She is calmer. She was never severely hyperactive, but her active behavior periods have come down a notch. She is able to concentrate and focus better. She can block out sounds and the background noise doesn't drown out what is going on in the foreground.

Candy still has some issues. She can see all the little details, but she doesn't get the big picture. That's the most significant one I guess. But she just keeps getting better. When I think about it, Candy might have been the kind of teenager to hurt herself. She might have started acting out had we not done what we did. Had we not put her through AIT and Tomatis, we might have had a child that we couldn't control. That thought keeps running through my mind. Had *The Davis Center* not been there to find the truth about my daughter and deal with it effectively, I don't know what kind of life I would have been facing with Candy.

STORY RESPONSE

Candy seemed to be a girl behind a mask when I first met her. She wanted to be included, but didn't always understand why. She didn't always fit in. She didn't want others to think she didn't get it, so she would sit quietly and just watch and listen (not always fully comprehending) and then make a remark about not caring about the conversation when she didn't get it. She also appeared scared at times.

When I first meet with parents, I offer a lot of information and since the human mind can only retain a small portion of what is presented, I know that most parents only zero in on those things that hit home for them. In Candy's case, her mother was able to identify with and put together many bits of information related to Candy's complex issues. Initially, I also try to prepare parents for all of the possible changes. In Candy's case, she started with wonderful positive changes and then when I began to address her core issues, Candy really regressed. She began to act like a little child at times. At one point, her mother reported that she was acting like a child from the country from which she was adopted. It was as though she was searching for or returning to her roots.

Candy's parents went through some difficult times while Candy was making change. At one point, I had to almost beg the mother not to stop the therapy. Since sound therapies make significant change, part of the process is like peeling back the layers of an onion. I keep peeling away, and more and more issues surface. The purpose is to identify and correct those poorly developed layers which affect all subsequent development. Such was the case with Candy. She needed to go back to early developmental stages so that she could move beyond those early stages that were holding her back. Once Candy got beyond the regressive stage, her mother said, "Thank you for making me carry on." Now Candy has a chance to really develop into a fine young lady.

Perhaps because Candy had been adopted, there seemed to be a bonding issue with her adoptive mother, even though she was a very loving, caring parent. Her mother reported in the story that their bond developed very strongly after the Tomatis method (a typical response), a very happy response for the entire family.

Candy's mother asked me about sensory integration. As with Matthew's story, sensory integration is a sign of issues that can be addressed via the voice-ear-brain connection. The therapies that are present on my "Tree" analogy help set the stage for better overall sensory integration reception from the world around us. The ear is more than a hearing mechanism. It is our balance center, our vestibular center, our proprioceptive center, and our muscle response center, all of which goes beyond the basics of being our hearing and listening center. The ear is so complex and the way sound stimulates the ear and the rest of the body through the ear is a major factor in how we view and respond to the world around us.

What's interesting about Candy's case is that so many professionals had not offered much help or hope. Educators did not seem to understand her uniqueness and were also unable to offer her a better way to learn. Even those schools reportedly knowledgeable about children with unique learning needs were unable to help. Few of the professionals linked the sense of hearing with listening in general, or with her demonstrated behaviors.

Candy's mother mentioned she noticed that using a quiet voice was helpful to Candy. This response is typically related to one type of hearing hypersensitivity. Candy's *DETP* verified and identified this special hypersensitivity, and therefore the first therapy she received addressed this hearing hypersensitivity. For some people, a muscle in the middle ear overreacts to sounds at very soft levels. By doing so, it allows too much sensation in both the cochlea and vestibular portions of the ear. After proper sound therapy, the muscle can relax and then the person can understand more of what is being said and therefore, tune in and respond better. Once retrained vocal loudness is no longer an issue.

Candy also began our *Read-Spell-Comprehend* program for a short time until finding a similar program closer to home. She managed to reach the level of the upper *Leaves and Branches* of *The Tree* analogy which finally allowed her to tackle some of her more difficult learning differences. She has continued to make good progress. Every few months, she does return for a Tomatis boost, so that she can continue to move forward. She will eventually reach the point where these boosts are no longer necessary. At that time, she may only wish to use sound therapy to enhance specific skill sets.

CHAPTER FOUR

Daniyal   ADHD, Adoption

> "He gets his homework done on his own. I don't have to ask him about it. He doesn't procrastinate. He used to drag a project on and wait until the last day. He doesn't do that anymore."

Randolph, New Jersey: Lilly holds her hands out as if she is holding a child and says with a smile in her eyes, "I have a happy little boy."

When I talk about my son Daniyal, I have some confusion. He isn't easy to categorize because he is so many different things all at once.

Daniyal was our first adopted child. From the beginning, I noticed many special things about him. Daniyal did everything before schedule. He was walking at eleven-months. He was fully potty trained by 2-years old. But there was something that didn't seem in place. He didn't develop language until later on. He was between eighteen- and twenty-months when he started speaking. Yet when he did, he spoke in full grammatically correct sentences. He wouldn't say, "I want water." He would say, "I want a glass of water." He wouldn't use childish language like, "I have to go potty." He would say, "I have to go to the bathroom."

By 2½-years old, Daniyal was having sensible, interesting conversations. He got along great with adults, engaging us in talks about things that were mature and interesting. He was very objective and always noticed things, and he was always so polite. A straight forward kid, he doesn't lie, cheat or steal. Even in his polite manner, he speaks his mind. I noticed how his honesty worked for him.

I remember taking Daniyal to Burger King one time. He had ordered a cheeseburger without pickles. But the cook forgot and placed pickles on Daniyal's cheeseburger anyway. He tapped the clerk on the hand and softly said, "I said I didn't want pickles." It was firm and assertive, but polite. It was from those kinds of instances that I never thought he would have problems with his social skills, but he did.

His honesty could also work against him. He didn't know how to manipulate or properly assess a situation. It's hard to explain, but most kids can walk into a room and know how they are supposed to act or what is expected of them. They can easily decide what to do and what not to do. Whether it is to be cool, popular, the teacher's pet or whatever they are attempting to be, most kids can figure out what will work for them in different cases. Daniyal couldn't quite work it like other kids.

He was diagnosed with ADHD at 5-years old. There was no support from the school system because Daniyal was so intelligent. I took him to a neurologist who put him on several medications, some of which were Ritalin and Adderall® *. These drugs are normally given to people with ADHD and those who also demonstrate behaviors like climbing the walls or jumping on furniture. The thing about Daniyal is he didn't climb the walls or jump on furniture. He wasn't destructive in the classroom. He didn't have temper tantrums all the time. I always wondered if he had been misdiagnosed.

At the time, I had been working as virologist, which is someone who studies and works with viruses. I quit my job so I could stay home and become available for teachers in case they would call or need me to come to the school. Sometimes, I would just drop into the school to take Daniyal out for lunch. He wasn't getting along too well with classmates and I thought getting him away for lunch could help give him a break. It was my way of helping because I had noticed that my son couldn't deal with

* Adderall is manufactured and distributed by Shire US Inc.

crowded places. He absolutely hated sudden noises. When we would have a family function like a wedding or something, Daniyal would greet everyone and then quickly disappear. He loved eating out, but he just couldn't handle large restaurants.

When Daniyal was about 8-years old, Alia was adopted into the family. Daniyal had been the only child in the household up to this point. Daniyal's first reactions were of jealousy. The attention he was used to getting was now being shared with an 18-month old girl. As they started growing up together, Daniyal would take things from his sister. He would try to hurt her when they played together. One of his favorite things was giving her noogies, rubbing his knuckles against the top of her head. Normally a noogie is dealt out in play, but Daniyal was serious when he did it to Alia. Daniyal would even throw toys at her. It was the first time I had ever seen Daniyal act this way. He had always been polite to others, but he was becoming quite a different person.

One day, we made a trip to Chinatown in New York City. I remember trying to hold Daniyal and Alia by the hand. They were on both sides of me. I looked down to see why they wouldn't hold my hand and something struck me a little funny. Alia was holding her nose because Chinatown smelled. Daniyal was holding his ears because it was too loud. I immediately thought of, "See no evil, hear no evil." Only in this case, it was, "Smell no evil, hear no evil."

Daniyal started to develop some problems in school. He was loud and he talked excessively. He never worked well on teams or in classroom groups. Kids didn't want him on their team or helping with their projects because he would mess them up or he just wouldn't do the work. After looking at things more closely, it seemed that it wasn't that Daniyal would not pay attention, it was just too bothersome. Sometimes the classroom would become too overwhelming for Daniyal to handle. In larger classrooms, he would hear everything in addition to what the teacher was saying. He could hear the hum of the light fixtures and the fluttering of a bird's wings outside the window. It would bother him. He didn't do his work. He would move around in class.

Even though he had developed some strong social skills, he was lacking in others. He was extra sensitive to criticism and was notorious for taking comments out of context. As other kids tend to do, they would instigate as if they loved seeing him get in trouble. He didn't understand how to deal with that. He couldn't just walk away or ignore it. He didn't have the ability to come back with witty comments of his own. Out of frustration, he would lash out negatively. Teachers have observed him touching and pushing other kids. I eventually had to sign Daniyal up for social skills classes and put him in group psychotherapy sessions. These were for behavior modification and to help Daniyal understand the consequences for his actions.

With all the noises he was hearing and the other kids instigating, he would desperately feel the urge to leave the classroom, although teachers wouldn't allow him. This would cause him to lash out in defense. In gym class, he acted up frequently and he absolutely refused to participate. Gym class was a given "A" and my son didn't want it. It wasn't as if he actually had to throw a ball. As long as he was trying to throw the ball, he would get an "A". The only thing I could think of was that it was very crowded and noisy. Gym class tends to be very hot, which just makes it even more miserable.

I was trying to work with the school, but they weren't willing to place him in specialized classes. Daniyal was too bright to be classified in school as someone with issues requiring more specialized attention than the mainstream students. I could never get the school to consider him for remedial classes because he had an above average IQ. He could do the work and get the lesson when he tried. I was sure the setting was the problem, not the class work.

When he started acting up and constantly getting into trouble, I was finally able to convince the school that there were some deeper issues. At 8-years old, I was able to get the school to classify Daniyal as ADHD with emotional problems so that I could get him into smaller classes with more specialized attention. His main classes were held in a smaller center. He would intermingle with other students for the rest of the day. He did well in small settings and would pick up quickly on academics.

I hadn't stopped looking for solutions. Everywhere I went, I was asking questions. I was pumping every professional I came into contact with to learn more about ADHD and to find out if my son actually fit that diagnosis. I finally found what I needed in a magazine. These were free magazines distributed throughout the township. Ordinarily they're passed out in pediatrician offices and libraries. Anywhere a parent might benefit from reading one. One day, I happened to be flipping through one and I found an advertisement about *The Davis Center*.

Thinking that my son had displayed sensitivity to loud noises and large crowds, the advertisement struck me as something I might want to pursue. I was not aware of sound-based therapies. When I told Daniyal's teachers about it, the school was not aware that it existed. My pediatrician was not aware of it. I always stressed that he was hypersensitive to noise and touch, but no one picked up on it. Fortunately I have an aggressive pediatric neurologist who had heard about it. He had sent other children to

The Davis Center, but they were autistic. He never made the connection between ADHD and sound-based therapies as a possible solution.

I decided to check it out. Daniyal was thirteen at the time. I called *The Davis Center* and set up an appointment. We did the *Diagnostic Evaluation for Therapy Protocol* and then we had a conference. Dorinne discovered many things from the test results. Specifically, she pointed to different things on the chart that were produced from the Listening Test and explained that the sound waves weren't going the way they were supposed to be going. They were always above or below the point where they were supposed to be.

After reviewing his *DETP*, Dorinne suggested Daniyal receive BioAcoustics first. I didn't see any change at all. Dorinne urged me that it would help in the long run even though you may see nothing at first and that this method would help lay the foundation for improvement overall. We were able to do BioAcoustics at home. They had programmed the sounds at *The Davis Center* and Daniyal would listen to them through headphones. I was concerned about the reason that BioAcoustics didn't seem to work. I also took to heart that it would work regardless of the fact that I was seeing no immediate results. Dorinne explained that it worked at a cellular level.

Daniyal was put through Auditory Integration Training next and we still didn't see any changes. Actually, Daniyal was getting tired of it. He went through it, but we could see his lack of interest. After AIT, there was a lapse for a couple of weeks. Then we put him in the first opening for Tomatis. We did a two week session. Dorinne recommended that we put Daniyal through a second session two months later.

At the start of the second session, I stopped Daniyal's medication. I wanted to give him one medication free summer. After his second session, I noticed some real changes finally. He became more compliant. He was much calmer about things. He didn't seem so stressed about everything. He wasn't so aggressive. He was even eating better. I had a happy little boy. One day, he mentioned to Dorinne that he was feeling different. He couldn't say exactly how, just that he felt something different.

This year of school is the best year he has had. His behavior is under control. He is interested in academics. He got some bad grades, but he understood he had to work harder. He said himself, "I know what I have to do now to get a better grade." So many things were improving with him. He hadn't shown much care about his grades or consequences before. But he was starting to care about what his future would be like. That's a true manifestation that the consequences of his actions were becoming more important to him. Despite the problems he had been having in school throughout the years, he is making plans to go to college.

I am no longer getting notes or e-mails about his behavior. He won a "Higher Achievement" award one month for overall academics and behavior. It's hard to explain exactly, I just see more maturity and a calmer presence about him. He gets his homework done on his own. I don't have to ask him about it. He doesn't procrastinate. He used to drag a project on and wait until the last day. He doesn't do that anymore.

When he started his third session of Tomatis, the lines on his Listening Test had finally closed. This was what we were hoping would happen. Dorinne found it unusual. When we talked, Dorinne knew something was bothering Daniyal, but she couldn't figure out this one little glitch in his hearing. She was able to figure it out and even pinpointed a timeframe. Dorinne knew that something had happened to Daniyal around the age of eight. Dorinne suggested that Daniyal had an issue he couldn't resolve. When I thought about it, I realized this was around the time Alia was introduced into the family. How she knew about that I don't know, but it was eye opening.

When Dorinne noticed that the curve on the Listening Test finally closed, she mentioned it to me. It was when Daniyal and Alia had finally become true brother and sister. They were closer and they were acting like they really loved each other. They still fight, but like normal siblings. He reads to her. He lets her play on his video games. He is very protective of her. He tries to take care of her like when we are getting ready to go somewhere, Daniyal will ask, "Where are your gloves?" They might fight over the amount of candy they get, when getting candy at the store, but he always gets her some.

Being more adjusted has really affected everything about Daniyal. He is more focused in school and he wants more out of it. He is calmer when he takes criticism from other kids. He is more into his sister and his family than he ever was. We were finally able to put the IQ with the person who fits it. Without *The Davis Center*, I'm not sure where Daniyal would be.

STORY RESPONSE

I first met Daniyal with his mother and his aunt, a teacher of special needs children. People often visit with me to determine if what I say makes sense. After asking many questions that first visit, his aunt left believing in the possibilities for positive change for Daniyal. I saw that Daniyal had a great deal of difficulty expressing what he was thinking and when he couldn't discuss something, a wall went up and he either gave up or acted inappropriately.

Daniyal's mother asked me if I help people with ADHD, as that was Daniyal's diagnosis. As I explain to all potential clients, I no longer say that I address any diagnoses. It isn't the diagnosis that I help. I now say that I help only those who demonstrate sound processing issues as evidenced by my *DETP*. It is the body's response to sound that is important to me. The tests that I perform are the only way for me to determine whether any sound therapy is appropriate for someone. When more than one therapy is appropriate, it will determine the correct order for their administration and is the key to successful treatment.

Daniyal was a young man who wanted to be liked by others, but didn't know how to go about it. His body's responses differed from what he wanted and his actions were inappropriate at times. Daniyal knew he was intelligent, but was frustrated with why he was unable to accomplish what his friends, who were less intelligent, seemed to accomplish with ease. This complicated and added to his self doubt. During his therapy, it was exciting to watch him blossom emotionally. He started to share feelings and emotions better. He demonstrated an ability to control some of his negative reactions and he learned more appropriate interactions with his peers. His sense of humor also evolved.

The *DETP* indicated the need for BioAcoustics first, followed by AIT. His mother reported no noticeable change during these two therapies. However, as I mentioned earlier, the essential foundation for positive change was being established by his body. This can be compared to the construction of a building. Only the ones with the firm foundation will support the building for many years. Daniyal could have made change from just Tomatis, but with the firmer foundation, the change is magnified and the body is better able to support the positive change over time.

Daniyal also received assistance with *The Davis Center's Read-Spell-Comprehend* program while doing Tomatis. This program helps build on auditory, visual, and language foundational reading and learning skills. He was prepared for this program, which is at the top of the *Leaves and Branches* of *The Tree*, because his foundation had been established.

Daniyal is a smart young man who will do well. He better understands who he is now and is making plans for his own future. Somewhere down the road, he may benefit from an additional Tomatis session as a "booster", but this would only be if he begins to notice that things could be better. There are hierarchies to the therapies because the system works like the peeling of an onion. It is important to peel away many layers of unorganized learning and development, so that these poorly developed layers can be stimulated, enhanced, modified, and challenged so that growth can occur. I was only able to identify the impact that Alia had on Daniyal around age 8, after a few layers had been peeled away. This major issue only surfaced after his many other layers were dealt with. Daniyal is now a much happier young man. He understands his actions and consequences better. It is a pleasure to see because now he can share the real Daniyal with everyone.

CHAPTER FIVE

Patrick

> "I feel like a great wonderful thing is happening to me.
> I feel like a real live boy."

Hackettstown, New Jersey: Wanda crosses her legs and clears her throat just before reaching for her cup of coffee.

Patrick was always uncomfortable with eye contact, he had a short attention span and we had to pull words out of him. He couldn't answer who, what, when, where, or how questions. One of the odd things about Patrick is when we would ask him a question, we became increasingly aware that it would take about ten seconds at least for his brain to register the question. We could see him working on it. We knew he had heard it. After it registered, then we knew that he had to think about the answer. Then he had to decide if he wanted to answer the question. We could see his wheels turning, but he wasn't saying anything. Also, Patrick thought we could read his mind. Saying things verbally didn't make sense to him. If he was screaming or crying, he wouldn't tell us what hurt or what was bothering him.

Playing with kids on the playground was something Patrick just didn't do. He wouldn't play on the swings or hang out at the playground. I didn't really understand at first what that was all about. I thought it was his social skills. He wouldn't look anyone in the eye and he wouldn't talk. So he couldn't play with kids very well. Patrick was in his own world. He just didn't connect to ours very well.

It wasn't just his talking; it was his hearing as well. Music bothered his ears greatly. If we ever took him to a park with a carousel, Patrick wouldn't want to ride on it. He would run away and put his hands over his ears. When the alarms at the firehouse would sound, Patrick would cover his ears and start screaming. He also did that during fire drills at school. He needed to be escorted to the exits while he was holding his ears and screaming. When they had assemblies at school, Patrick would have to leave the room. It was too loud with all those students in one room and it would overwhelm Patrick to the point that he just couldn't handle it.

When Patrick was first diagnosed with autism at age 2, I started reading everything I could find. One good book that comes to mind is *The Sound of a Miracle* by Annabel Stehli. It's a book about a mother who put her child through the Auditory Integration Training. Ms. Stehli published a sequel called *Dancing in the Rain*. It is a compilation of stories about people who have gone through AIT. I found a center in New York City that did AIT. Although back then, Patrick was out of control and going to New York City just didn't appeal to me. I was so overwhelmed with the new information that Patrick was autistic. I had him placed in a special needs class where they taught basic things. I wanted more for him, so I put him in a school for autistic children. After two years I saw little improvement.

Frustrated, I began to look for other solutions. I found an article in the paper about children with autism. It said something like, "Do you or your child have learning disabilities, ADD or autism?" Well, that caught my eye. It was about a seminar at *The Davis Center*. *The Davis Center* was only 15-minutes away, much more appealing than going all the way to New York City. I signed Patrick up for the initial assessment of the *Diagnostic Evaluation for Therapy Protocol* that night, anticipating the need for AIT.

I really didn't come to the center with high expectations. I wasn't sure anything was going to work. But I thought if it changes anything for the better, it is money worth spending. I would pay a million dollars just for Patrick to talk to me, just to have a conversation with him.

With the *DETP* complete, Patrick's plan was mapped out. Dorinne suggested we start with AIT, which we did in June. Patrick was 8, but he would be turning 9-years old within a month. They conducted a hearing sensitivity test before, during and after therapy. They put headphones on him and he listened to music. Patrick's hearing was so off the wall. He was really sensitive to sound when he first started.

Patrick was put in a sound treated room which had a chair and a table with some books on it. They placed headphones on him and he listened for a half an hour. Through the headphones, he would be listening to Stevie Wonder one day and then to some New Age music the next day. It was ordinary music, but it sounded like a radio station that wasn't quite tuned in correctly. It was like the music was staticky and other sounds were embedded. The sound would be in the left-ear and then it would fade and transfer between ears. Patrick would listen for half an hour in the morning and another half an hour in the afternoon. At first, he screamed and cried when they put the headphones on him. Patrick loved Sponge Bob, so I bought him a Sponge Bob toy and told him that he could only have it while the headphones stayed on his head.

Something happened after the first day of AIT. On the way home, Patrick reached over and took my hand. He started playing with my hair. He had never initiated contact with me. This was the first time.

After just one week of having completed AIT, we went to the park. I was sure how Patrick was going to act because there was a carousel. The music had always bothered him and Patrick would run away holding his ears. Patrick didn't run away this time. When the carousel started turning, Patrick ran beside the carousel. He was smiling and enjoying it.

Patrick started playing with the kids on the playground. He was more of a kid. When we got home, he wanted to go back to the playground. He ran to the swings and jumped on one. He would play with the other kids. When the fire alarm sounded at the fire house, I thought I would have to cover Patrick's ears. But he was fine. It bothered him a little, and then he turned to me and started to tell me what it was all about. "The cat got caught in the tree. They got in the fire engine and drove where the tree was. The cat said 'Meow...I'm stuck in the tree'. The firemen went and got the cat. The cat said 'Meow' again and that meant thanks." That was the first time Patrick told a story. I didn't have to pull it out of him. He was excited to tell me about it.

At the end of AIT, when Patrick went back to summer school, the teachers noticed the difference. There was a fire drill. Patrick didn't scream. He left like everyone else. During the assemblies, Patrick normally had to leave the room because it was too loud. He no longer had to leave the assembly.

I forgot to mention earlier that Patrick had problems with some of his motor skills too. His upper body had no muscle tone. Patrick loved Sponge Bob and Sponge Bob had this thing with holding up his pinky. Patrick couldn't do that. He would have to hold up his index finger instead because he couldn't hold up just his pinky. After that first week of AIT, Patrick was watching the Sponge Bob cartoon and Patrick was able to hold up his pinky like Sponge Bob.

Patrick was quite a different kid now. Before, when he was crying or screaming, he wouldn't tell anyone what hurt or what the problem was. He could tell people now. He was initiating conversations. He could answer the Who, What, When, Where, Why and How questions. When I asked him who was in the room, he could tell me. When I asked him what the book he was reading was all about, he wanted to tell me. One time, I asked him what he wanted for dinner. He answered, "Macaroni and cheese." After dinner, he brought his plate over to the table. I asked him if he wanted to go swimming. Patrick said, "Yes." He answered me. He looked me in my eyes and answered my question, on the second day of therapy.

We did AIT for two weeks and immediately afterwards started Tomatis. Then we waited a month and did Tomatis for two more weeks. They did a Listening Test on Patrick to determine at each frequency the point where Patrick interprets the sounds heard through air and sound perceived by bone. They do a Listening Test before and the after each therapy session. The Listening Test produces a chart that Dorinne reads to determine Patrick's listening posture. The lines on the chart should touch. Patrick's lines weren't touching at all.

During Tomatis, there was a 3-year old child and a 70-year old lady in the room with Patrick. There was a trampoline for kids to jump on. They could even sleep if they wanted. They could do anything as long as they kept the headphones on their heads. During Tomatis they played filtered Mozart music. The staff at *The Davis Center* gave me homework to do everyday. I had to write down everything that was new and improved about Patrick. After only a few days, I had some pretty full pages, as he had made so many improvements. Patrick started with so many things wrong with him; there was no way he would not be able to improve.

I didn't have to give Patrick the Sponge Bob for him to keep the headphones on his head this time. Patrick was excited about going to *The Davis Center*. Something was happening in his head that was good. He didn't know how to explain it or what it was, but it was just something good. Patrick had been going to an art therapist for about six or seven years. Her name was Belinda. She had a computer where he would write things. She used it for him to communicate with her. One day, he wrote, "I feel like a great wonderful thing is happening in me. I feel like a real live boy."

The Listening Test after the second session of Tomatis was showing some very good results. The lines were almost touching and had crossed over five times. That was explained to me as a good thing. Patrick is supposed to finish his last session within a month and his Listening Test should be completely in line by then.

The one thing about all this is how lonely it all feels. Other parents look at you like you're crazy when you're explaining what is going on with your child. You feel alone thinking your child is one of a kind and no one can relate, but my child wasn't the only child going through this.

One day, when Patrick had finished the first session of Tomatis, there was another parent of a 6-year old boy. The boy was screaming. He was an autistic child too and he did not want to go in *The Davis Center*. I walked up to the mother and gave her stickers. I told her it would work. The boy settled down a little. Then I said to her, "Don't worry about your child yelling and screaming. *The Davis Center* sees it all the time. Your son is going to improve. Just go on in there and don't worry. Things will get better."

I remember her look. It was a look of wonder like how could you possibly know how I'm feeling. The special need seems so rare that parents don't realize that there are other parents dealing with the same thing. We always feel like we're alone in the world. The bonding makes us feel pretty good.

STORY RESPONSE

When I first met Patrick, he was 8½-years old. He had been adopted at birth. Sometimes adopted children have special bonding issues. Patrick's issue went far beyond bonding. He was also diagnosed with autism. Initially, Patrick overreacted to everything. He was extremely fearful at his initial assessment and seemed fearful of the slightest unknown.

His *DETP* suggested that he needed AIT first, followed by Tomatis. BioAcoustics was suggested as a possible third therapy only if the outcomes hoped for by the end of Tomatis were not achieved. A BioAcoustics voiceprint would be redone after Tomatis to determine the need for this therapy. To date, Patrick has done very well without adding the BioAcoustics piece. He will continue to be monitored, though, to determine if this therapy may still be the missing piece of his puzzle.

It is easy to confuse all the various sound-based therapies. It is also easy to confuse the names of the therapies as well as what each does. For example, Patrick's mother originally thought that Annabel Stehli's daughter went to a school in New York City for AIT. Actually, she received AIT with Dr. Bérard, the creator of the method, in France. She came back to New York and was then able to go to a school in New York, but did not receive the therapy there. Patrick's mother searched for the school in New York and found one for Patrick, which she mentions in her story.

Others confuse Tomatis and AIT, and it is not uncommon for some practitioners to also confuse these two therapies. In fact, some people consider the therapies the same. They are definitely not the same; they are distinctly different. They work at different levels as explained by my protocol *The Tree of Sound Enhancement Therapy*. AIT represents the *Root System* and Tomatis, the *Trunk* of *The Tree*.

When evaluating how a person functions initially, understanding the difference between these two therapies can mean the difference between a "miracle" change and just a regular change.

I'll never forget one special day that Patrick came to the office during his therapy. His mother was so excited to tell me what he had written for his art therapist—that "he felt like a real live boy." I sat back and thought about the child that Patrick had been hiding inside before therapy, simply because he could not process sound appropriately. He now has so much to offer. Can you imagine what it is like to view the world from a stilted perspective, trying in every way possible to fit in, while your body won't let you? Patrick was not able to fit in. He is now a happier boy since receiving the therapies. What must it have been like to not have a friend, nor know how to be one, until age 9!

Patrick now enjoys living with sound in comfort. He is no longer over stimulated because his ear is able to stabilize all of his sensory input. Most people do not realize that our ear is our major sensory stimulator. All of our senses are stimulated through the ear by sound vibration.

You may also notice that I discuss "sound processing" not auditory processing, a term frequently used by audiologists, physicians, and educators. Auditory processing typically relates to processing for communication purposes as it relates to speech and language. However, sound processing encompasses much more. It is because of how the body processes sound stimulation that the positive changes occur using sound-based therapies as I incorporate them into my concept *The Tree of Sound Enhancement Therapy.*

Patrick's mother relates how much calmer life is now that Patrick can fit in better. Having moved to New Jersey and having found *The Davis Center*, she feels the move was meant to be as both her and her son's lives have changed so dramatically.

CHAPTER SIX

Robbie   Autism, Hyperacousis

> "Amazingly, he started talking more. He started singing.
> He now sings songs I never knew he knew.
> He loves music. He is a much happier child."

Boise, Idaho: While rubbing her hands together, Sharon begins her story after thoughtful deliberation.

obbie was born happy, healthy and normal. When he was six months old, we moved from New Jersey to Texas. When I stopped nursing, I noticed that he was allergic to the the normal formula. So I put him on a soy formula and he started developing earaches. He had ear infections for almost a year. They had him on antibiotics, but they were afraid to take him off of them when the infections cleared. He was on antibiotics for a solid six months.

He got another ear infection while still on the antibiotics, so they recommended putting tubes in his ears. This all happened before he was even 1-year old. He didn't get any more infections after that, although that's when other things started happening. He used to be able to say "Momma" and "Dadda". Then he stopped all language. Between the ages of thirteen- and fifteen-months, he started clapping his hands and he wouldn't even make eye contact. When people would come into the house, he would run upstairs and I would find him hiding underneath his crib. He started to play with toys in unusual ways, like he became fixated on rocks and marbles, even dirt. He loved watching the dirt drop in front of his eyes—all these unusual behaviors are called stimming as he does it to stimulate himself. Another "stim" he enjoyed was crumbling everything, especially a sandwich. He would just make it into crumbs.

His daily actions became more unusual. He stopped sleeping and started running through the hallways upstairs, just back and forth, back and forth. At first, I thought maybe he needed to burn up energy. Or maybe he was going to be a track star or something. By 18-months, I definitely knew something was wrong with him. His bizarre behavior and loss of language were continually escalating.

I took him to the pediatrician and they said that he was a normal boy with ear infections. They went with what they knew and told me things like, "He might not be able to hear. That's why he's not responding to you." They told me that boys develop slower anyway. They just tied it all into the ear infections, but they weren't really concerned at all. And it wasn't just one particular doctor. It was a group of them. No one showed the least little bit of concern that the problem could be anything else.

We decided to start early intervention on our own. A therapist came to the house. They basically just played with him on the floor and diagnosed him as "gravitationally insecure." They explained that as not knowing where his body is in space. All the people I have asked or talked to about his gravitationally insecure condition have been stumped by the diagnosis. No one has ever heard of it.

We made an appointment with a hearing specialist because we thought he was deaf. Nothing made sense to me. I was just grasping at straws. So, we made the appointment and they did a hearing test. The test is called a brainstem auditory evoked response or BAER test. They actually put electrodes on his head and they were able to tell if he is able to hear without him responding to sounds or questions. We had to come back a second time because the sedatives they tried to give him made his actions more turbulent rather than putting him to sleep. When we took him back the second time, they told us there was nothing wrong with his hearing.

We made an appointment with a developmental pediatrician. By this time Robbie was two and a half. The waiting period to see this special pediatrician was six months. However, we never made it to the pediatrician because we moved back to New Jersey. We did that mainly because there wasn't a good support network for us and no one was really helping. I wasn't happy at all with what was happening. My husband worked it out with his company to make the move and we soon found ourselves back in New Jersey ready to see what could be done for Robbie there.

We took him to doctors. But, they weren't too alarmed. They asked me if I had placed Robbie in therapy. When I told them I did, they said that's all I could do. I had a feeling of helplessness. I was getting the same runaround in New Jersey that I got in Texas. I know there was more I could do, I just needed to find it.

We placed Robbie in a pre-school handicapped program that met for two and a half hours every day through the week. The program did nothing for him, and nothing we did worked. I would go in to watch him. He looked so odd and different compared to the other kids. Everyone would say things like, "Have you ever seen a child like this? I have never seen a child like him."

I mentioned these concerns to the pre-school teacher and finally she told me to talk to the psychiatrist. He handed me a test called the Childhood Autism Rating Scale or CARS. He told me to go home and fill it out. It's a test that puts your child on the spectrum to see if a child is autistic. I was thrown.

My husband had always suggested taking him to a school for autistic children and suggested Eden in the Princeton area. I would always get upset at the thought of it. In my mind, children like that bang their heads on walls. I was not going to stick him with those kids. I know my son is severe. I am not trying to paint a pretty picture in any way and maybe he would have done well there. But I am the only one he developed a strong connection with and I just couldn't think of him being diagnosed with autism.

When I started going through the questions in the CARS, I wasn't even half way through the test and I knew my child had autism. My heart sunk. But I had to finish the test and then score it. He scored on the severe end of the spectrum. This is when I went into overdrive. Now I knew what was wrong.

I made an appointment with the psychiatrist. It was very overwhelming. I was asking, "What does this mean?" The psychiatrist told me that I was in store for a lifelong journey and that there was nothing I could do. I asked about the schools that work with autistic children and the psychiatrist kept telling me to forget about it. He said I would never get Robbie into one. I kept repeating to him that I had to try, "I can't just say it's over already." He urged me to wait until Robbie became five and we could talk about it again. "We'll revisit this and see where we are," is what he said. He wanted me to keep Robbie in the pre-school handicap program.

They were keeping Robbie strapped in a chair because they couldn't control him. They were using the chair that is supposed to be used for a child with physical problems whose muscles aren't physically capable of providing the proper support. Robbie didn't need that. They were using it because they couldn't control him. I thought he looked worse in school. I couldn't believe how much worse he was getting.

At the time, I wasn't aware that the district would have to pay for the school if Robbie were found in need of it. Now that Robbie had a proper diagnosis of autism, the school system was supposed to provide proper therapy to constantly keep him engaged. A doctor by the name of Ivar Lovaas founded the Lovaas Institute and began an intensive behavioral therapy on a group of children. That therapy has come to be known as Applied Behavior Analysis or ABA. This is what the school is supposed to follow. My heart sunk further because I trusted this school psychiatrist with my child's life and he was only making decisions from a money standpoint.

One day, my mother-in-law handed me a book called *The Sound of a Miracle* by Annabel Stehli. It was from that book that I had heard of a certain therapy that had cured a girl with autism. I started looking for the therapy and I found Dorinne. I was surprised that the place was in New Jersey. But when we brought him in to do the Auditory Integration Training, his autistic behaviors kept him from sitting still. He was so out of control, he wouldn't sit or keep the headphones on his head. I was allowed to touch him and that would calm him down a bit. But I couldn't do that the whole time. I knew this wasn't going to work. I just couldn't handle it at that time.

My daughter came with us and she also had language and behavioral issues. Her articulation was so bad and she was placed in the special education program. *Hear You Are*, Dorinne's company before *The Davis Center*, tested her and we put her through AIT. We didn't see much of a change. Dorinne had told us that there might be little if no change. I wanted to do it anyway because I wanted to help her. However, I stopped the therapy, because I felt like I had given it a try and saw little change, so I pulled her out.

I started calling all the schools that specialize in autism. In my searches, I found a real guardian angel, a consultant in the field of autism. She took me under her wing and told me so many things. She evaluated Robbie as a professional. She told me Robbie needed to be in a full-time program. He needed speech therapy and Applied Behavior Analysis using discrete trials. She said I couldn't wait. I had to start immediately. Through her connections, she got us into an outreach therapy program. They worked with Robbie six hours a week. I told the consultant what was going on at the school and she said I couldn't settle for that. I had to let the school know I wanted better. I had to demand more from the school. When I told her about Robbie being strapped to the chair, she said that was inexcusable. I needed to stand up for my son.

I confronted the district that what they were doing was not appropriate. The next time I went into the school and found him still strapped to the chair, I wrote them a letter. They dragged their feet. I told them I wanted to apply to send Robbie to a private school. They refused and I hired an attorney. I felt like I couldn't waste another day. I had already wasted enough time. I wouldn't stop and I went faster than the district was ready, which was probably good because it threw them off balance. I would visit the school and watch them. I would take notes and document everything. But obviously, I couldn't disrupt the class or interfere with anything. They were trying to tell me that the teacher who was there was an expert with autism. That just wasn't true.

I don't want to blame the teacher at all. She was placed in the situation by the district. They were telling her to tell me that she could handle the situation and that Robbie didn't need any more than what the school was willing to provide. I honestly think she would have given me anything I wanted, but the district was only giving her so much to provide for her students.

I also hired another expert from another school that wasn't Eden. I wanted to have him evaluate the school Robbie was attending to prove that what they were providing wasn't appropriate. The district didn't want me to do this, but they couldn't stop me either. The expert would take three weeks. The district started to panic and asked for mediation. I agreed and then within a day or two, mediation wasn't working. We couldn't agree on anything. So I called my lawyer and told the district I would give them a court date. I had a court date at around the same time the expert was about to come in to have a look at things. I was moving so fast that I don't think they really had time to get their thoughts together. The district decided to get together and settle. They agreed to create a full autism program and hire an experienced teacher. They were going to create a summer program and they hired a one-on-one teacher for Robbie to give him five hours of attention a day. In addition, by March they had agreed to hire a therapist to work one-on-one with Robbie, but they were trying to get the full program up and running by September. The teacher that they finally did hire had twenty-years of experience. The therapist who had been there couldn't help Robbie, but the new teacher was wonderful. When she came on board, everything changed in our lives.

I was coming in very hesitantly and the new teacher had already been warned about me. "This crazy mother who is very difficult…" The new teacher was very understanding and had great patience with families. She told me that I could come in and watch and do anything I wanted. So I started to come in to volunteer at first. She started training me. I wasn't there daily, but I was there three times a week. She taught me so much to help Robbie. In just the first six months, I was getting a child back. It was amazing how the right type of treatment began to make change. The most important thing that she ever taught me was positive reinforcement. It works so much better than negative. It helped me to be a better mother to all of my children.

For the following years, he would get occupational therapy. We did the gluten and casein free diet, which is a common diet for people with autism. We did vitamin therapy, speech therapy, the full day autism program, the summer program. We did it all.

At around age 10½, we also did neural feedback. We did it as a pilot study. It was offered to see if it was going to help children with autism. I saw some changes. He seemed happier and he started getting independent skills. Little, but there were some changes.

We attended a conference about autism. While I was standing there talking to the neural feedback person, Dorinne joined the conversation. Dorinne started talking about Tomatis and so I went over to her booth. I was in awe by what I saw. I decided that Robbie was now able to go through it. It was time. He would fit and be able to do it. But first, Dorinne had us start with the *Diagnostic Evaluation for Therapy Protocol*. Once again, AIT was his starting place.

During AIT, Robbie seemed like he heard more noises and sounds. His language started to increase. He was more aware of his surroundings. He did show signs of discomfort at times. He would struggle a little when the sounds seemed to hurt him. We stuck it out and held him and massaged him. I guess he never was aware, but all of a sudden he was noticing birds and planes. Even though he wasn't deaf, he couldn't hear certain sounds. I noticed that although he hadn't been hearing these things, he could hear them now.

Now that this new world was opening up for Robbie and he was more aware of everything around him, he was getting fearful.

He would panic at times because we had put him in a world he never knew existed. It took about a year to get through most of his fears. With autism, there are many compulsive behaviors and repetitive behaviors. What started as a fear became a compulsive behavior. The fear triggered the behavior, but then it had nothing to do with the fear and just turned into a pattern or a compulsive behavior. For instance, he would hear a sound that would come from outside and it would cause him to become fearful of going outdoors. After awhile it wasn't about the fear anymore. He was over the issues with the sounds, but he still didn't want to go outside.

Immediately after AIT, within a week, he started Tomatis. Dorinne told us that it would be beneficial to keep going. Tomatis blew our socks off. It was so unbelievable from a physical standpoint. He had been very thin with dark circles under his eyes. During Tomatis, he wanted more food. He gained weight and became nice and plump like a little boy should be. His skin had been pasty. When he started eating better, his skin became more natural in color and he just started looking healthier. He also started sleeping more soundly through the night.

So many other things started happening to him. Amazingly, he started talking more. He started singing. He now sings songs I never knew he knew. He loves music. He is a much happier child. He wants to be more with the family and he comes down to the family room to spend more time with us. And he initiates play with us. I am finally getting to really know my Robbie, and starting to see the real him. It's not just the child lost within his body. It's finally the real Robbie.

Sound therapies made his life more enjoyable, and when his life is more enjoyable, we all benefit. It makes our lives more enjoyable. Many parents I tell think I am crazy. They don't think all these changes are logical. The funny thing is I would have tended to agree. I keep saying, "I know it sounds crazy, but this is what happened. I know it doesn't make sense, but trust me it happened."

We spent years doing occupational therapy (OT) and speech therapy (ST) and we did see some changes and some improvement. But with sound-based therapies, I have seen much more change in the last year and a half than the ten years Robbie was doing OT and speech therapies. After Robbie made such great progress, we put our daughter Cassie through Tomatis. Cassie's changes weren't as dramatic because she is higher functioning. She made progress as well. She sings, she is happier, and she gets along with other kids better. She has better posture and walks better. She's older now, I can talk to her, and I can ask her how she feels. She tells us she doesn't feel any better, but my husband and I notice an overall well-being.

STORY RESPONSE

Robbie, who initially visited my first company, *Hear You Are*, was a fearful little boy, with numerous sensory issues. He was just lost within himself. His parents had difficulty dealing with "negative behaviors" because they feared adding to his rough times and they were having difficulty accepting a diagnosis of autism.

These responses were not unlike many of the parents I see. Many parents of autistic children decide to wait until the child can handle the therapies better before coming to me. This of course poses the question, what does the child have to go through to get to the stage where they can handle the therapies? For example, a child may not want to put headphones on because of not liking the sensation. This response is typically related to the connection of touch, sensation, and the ear. However, typically after a period of 4 days of therapy, the child no longer reacts to the headphones and actually enjoys himself because change has already occurred and the negative sensation has disappeared. Another example is that of the child with hearing hypersensitivities. Sound therapies take away these hypersensitivities. If the child has hypersensitivities at an early age and does not receive the remedial therapies until he can handle it better, say at age 6 or 7, he has had to deal with his hearing hypersensitivities for many years, exacerbating the responses and compounding the developmental delays over the years. By changing the hypersensitivities at an earlier age, the child has time to begin to settle into his new sound world, and begin to attempt better communication skills at an earlier age. The earlier therapeutic intervention can be initiated, the more positive the responses.

When I read Robbie's story that his school used to keep him strapped in a chair, and knowing how hypersensitive he was, I often think that Robbie was simply trying to get away from the noise around him by trying to move. His being strapped in creates a horrible picture in my mind, especially when I know that I can diminish his hypersensitivity.

When Robbie's parents took him out of AIT at my old company, they did him a disservice. The changes that had begun once he had started therapy were not allowed to fully develop. In reality, it should have started at an earlier age. His parents also took his sister out of therapy when it was first introduced, again not allowing for its effects to be established. With sound therapy, it is important to finish at least the basic programs. If not, the person can be left with unresolved issues and semi-developed skills that over time will diminish.

Robbie's mother also mentioned that they had taken him for other hearing tests and that the results were normal. Very often the people I see have normal hearing. In fact, I expect them to have normal hearing. Their issues typically stem from how they process sound stimulation—notice I did not say how they process auditory stimulation. There is a major difference between the two and it is one of the main reasons why a typical hearing test does not provide enough information for me diagnostically. The impact of sound stimulation goes way beyond auditory stimulation.

Robbie had also seen many specialists, including developmental pediatricians. It is not surprising that many of them did not refer to *The Davis Center*. Physicians have only recently begun to hear about the positive changes we make and are now referring patients to us. This is an exciting development, since in the past they would not refer clients because medical insurance would not cover some of the therapies. They would however, send family members for our sound therapy services.

As with most families with autistic children, the parents try any program or therapy. In my book *Sound Bodies through Sound Therapy*, I discuss how the ear and the voice-ear-brain connection are pivotal to the development of the child. During the development of the fetus, the ear is the only sensory system that is fully functioning. All the other sensory systems become fully functional at birth. This demonstrates that the natural development of the ear plays a major part of a child's overall development. If that is so, it follows that when looking at how the child develops, we should first look at the ear and the voice-ear-brain connection. When this is stabilized, other areas of development can be addressed with better success. This is why the term "Sensory Integration Dysfunction" became so important over the past few years and why occupational therapists and pediatricians are more aware of this as a developmental issue. Sensory integration is directly related to the voice-ear-brain connection. However, it only addresses one piece of the entire connection. So yes, small changes can occur, but change will occur more appropriately if all of the foundational connections are enhanced.

This same voice-ear-brain connection includes wellness and is an important part of the initial developmental process. My "Davis Addendum to the Tomatis Effect" demonstrates this wellness connection 100% of the time, and so not only must we look at learning developmentally, but also wellness developmentally.

Because of Robbie's age, fear of unknown sounds began to take hold and his parents finally returned, started, and completed AIT. His mother reported that he began to hear more noises and sounds. Because of his hearing hypersensitivities, Robbie had survived by shutting out the world (tuning out), which perpetuated and exacerbated the problem. After therapy, he became more aware of his surroundings and was able to hear new sounds. The world began to open up for Robbie. His brain finally adjusted to his new sense of hearing. He now responds to his name quickly and responds with some conversational interaction. He is happier and beginning to understand more about who he is and what he can do.

CHAPTER SEVEN

Jackson   ADHD

"It was absolutely tremendous. His reading comprehension got better. His ability to process what he heard got better. We would take him to the Rutgers basketball games and he started to respond to what they were saying over the loud speakers. That was something new."

Metuchen, New Jersey: Stacey has to interrupt the conversation to show the plumber where her leak is. She then focuses her thoughts on her son's story.

*J*ackson's birth came a little ahead of time. I had high blood pressure so I was on bed rest. His birth was induced a week early. It was rough. I pushed him for three and a half hours and Jackson ended up being delivered with forceps. After that, everything was pretty normal. He developed normally. He wasn't a real chatty kid, but he learned to speak at an average rate.

Jackson liked it when I read to him. He enjoyed the closeness and the cuddling. He always liked to draw and he is very good at it. He loves colors and designs, and has always had an eye for beauty. My neighbor had a stained glass window on the way upstairs to her bedrooms. It was hard keeping him away from that window. It was on a landing that went upstairs. He was just a toddler so we were afraid he was going to fall and hurt himself. But once we brought him downstairs, he was right back up to that window again.

When he was about two and a half, he went from a crib to a big boy bed. The first day I came up to check on him, and he was sound asleep, but he had totally dismantled the whole thing. He used to do that everyday. I kept telling him that he couldn't keep taking his bed apart. But looking back on it, that was an early sign that he had a hyperactive personality. As far as processing goes, he didn't ask questions when I was reading to him. If I slowed down the reading, I would lose him. I subconsciously knew that I had to read fast or I would lose him. In fact, as Jackson was growing up, one of the things he used to say when I got into a long explanation about something, "Too many words, Mom."

When Jackson would try to tell you a story about something, he would start by telling you about a cat in the window and end up with something about a carnival. He was all over the place. It was because of these small things I was picking up on, that I had Jackson evaluated. The Department of Special Services in the school system evaluated him and told me that he had processing issues. Jackson was three and a half at the time. I sent Jackson to a private Speech Pathologist for about a year. She would work with Jackson on doing things in sequential order. She would have four pictures that Jackson would have to put in order of when something happened. Conversationally, she would work with Jackson staying on topic, rather than floating from one thing to another.

When Jackson was four and a half, we sent him to an early intervention program through the school system. They worked with him on pretty much the same things as his private Speech Pathologist. There were about ten kids in the class so they really got specialized attention. Jackson did great with all of this. We thought, "That's that." And it was for the most part.

In kindergarten, the only thing that Jackson had a problem with was staying on task. That was the biggest thing. Other than that, Jackson was fine. He was doing pre-reading, and spelling was coming along. I had a normal kid.

Then when first grade came along, the teacher noticed some issues with Jackson early in the school year. She would give the class an instruction, "Take out your math book and turn to page sixty." Jackson would be on the wrong page or he would be off task in some other way. The kids would laugh at him when he wasn't on task. Jackson got to the point where he wouldn't move a muscle. He didn't want that to happen anymore. So he wouldn't do anything. This didn't go over too well with the teachers. They started calling me and telling me everything that was happening. Jackson had other issues as well. The school hours were too long for him. He complained about that. He couldn't sit still in class. This is all part of his Attention Deficit Hyperactivity Disorder or ADHD. Although Jackson wasn't diagnosed with that until he was eight. So at the time, we didn't know he had these issues. From day one, his favorite subjects in school were gym and recess. In gym he could move around and be active, plus he didn't have to focus on anything for too long of a time.

Jackson was frustrated in school and the teacher didn't understand why. If he was given an assignment to do with written instructions at the top, the teacher didn't understand why he couldn't do the instructions. The teacher was puzzled because he had been one of the few kids that started the school year able to read.

Over the summer, after first grade, I found The Listening Program, but it wasn't through *The Davis Center*. We put Jackson through it and we saw tremendous growth. He was able to articulate better. I was excited that The Listening Program had benefited him so well. Little did I realize that this was just one step in a long journey.

Second grade actually went pretty well. He had a wonderful teacher. Then third grade hit and he was back down to having difficulties. She was a good teacher, but what I am finding out about the school system is that they only teach to the general population. Anyone outside of the norm can get left behind very quickly. I didn't really know where to turn. Obviously, The Listening Program hadn't worked all that well. Jackson was starting to have difficulties again. I went online and found *The Davis Center*.

I was skeptical about it at first. I think that's natural with things that you find online, but there was nothing else. We were pretty impressed with Dorinne and had the initial testing done using the *Diagnostic Evaluation for Therapy Protocol*.

The first therapy Jackson did was AIT. It was during the third grade school year that Jackson went through AIT. I would pick him up at lunch and get his school work. *The Davis Center* was about an hour from our house. He would do his first AIT session. Then we would go to the library so he could get his homework done and return back for the second session and go home. We did this everyday for ten days.

Actually it was interesting, during AIT Jackson became chatty. This was new. He had never been one to respond to things like what was being said on the radio. But all of a sudden, he started to respond to things. If the announcer on the radio said something about the weather, Jackson would comment about it. "The weather tomorrow is going to be pretty bad mom." This was all new. He also started to become a bit less frustrated all the time. He had always had a very short fuse, but now he was doing better in that regard.

We went straight from AIT into Tomatis. I didn't pick him up at lunch. I waited until after school to do Tomatis. The difference was that he could sit there and do his homework while he was listening for some of the time. During AIT, he had been only allowed to sit and listen in a small room. During AIT he wasn't allowed to do anything for that half an hour.

When I would talk to his teacher at school, she referred to his sessions as "The Tomato" thing. She was very frustrating to work with. I gave her literature on everything Jackson was going through at *The Davis Center*. I don't think she read any of it. One of the major things was that Jackson should have been in the front row away from the windows and away from the heater. Before he started any of the sound therapies, he had a slight hearing sensitivity. I remember having to get Jackson ear plugs for the fire drills. Those fire drills would send him through the roof. Anyway, I talked to his teacher about his seating. One night during a teacher conference, I asked her where Jackson was seated and discovered he was in the back next to the windows and the radiator. It was the opposite of where he should have been. I just couldn't get any support from her at all.

The following summer, we put Jackson through the *Read-Spell-Comprehend* program. He made some gains. Anytime you have four hours a day, five days a week one-on-one time with a teacher, it can't be a bad thing. Jackson was not a morning person, and didn't take too well to the program at first. One day, I had to have a mom and son talk with him. I told him that one day he was going to thank me for this. And it was during the second week that Jackson started to come around and enjoy it. He looked at me one day and said, "OK, I'm enjoying it. But I'm not ready to thank you yet."

The *Read-Spell-Comprehend* program was what helped Jackson get through the fourth grade. I had told Jackson that if he worked hard through the *Read-Spell-Comprehend* program, he wouldn't have to struggle so much through school. I was getting smarter too. I started to keep a folder. Every time Jackson came home with a good grade, I would put it in his folder. Through all of this, Jackson started to think he was stupid. I set out to prove him wrong. When your child thinks he's stupid, it just breaks your heart. When Jackson would be doing homework and it would get a little difficult, he would start with, "I'm so stupid." I would pull out the folder and show him his good grades, "Is this the work of a stupid kid?"

One day, he asked me why he didn't get good grades last year. I reminded him of our conversation over the summer that if he worked hard, he would get good grades. He looked at me and said, "OK, but I'm still not ready to thank you yet."

Next Jackson did the Fast ForWord program series. All through the fourth grade, during the school year, Jackson did all three of the Fast ForWord programs, one after the other. It was absolutely tremendous. His reading comprehension got better. His ability to process what he heard got better. We would take him to the Rutgers basketball games and he started to respond to what they were saying over the loud speakers. That was something new. I think he had been tuning those things out all of this life.

His fourth grade teacher was very supportive of the Fast ForWord program and everything we were doing with Jackson at *The Davis Center*. When Jackson would come in and share something with her, she would get excited about it. It was just a great year.

To get ready for Jackson's summer, I took a Lindamood-Bell course so that I could work with Jackson myself on visualizing and verbalizing. I also sent a friend to take the On Cloud Nine math course. We worked with Jackson on those things over the summer. However fifth grade turned out to be a disaster. This was the first year that he had been in middle school, which means he was changing classes all day. Jackson loved it, but in his Individual

Education Plan (IEP), his teachers were supposed to use an FM system, where they wear a portable microphone. Jackson was supposed to have a headset on so that he could hear his teachers better. The FM system filters out background noise. It turned out that the school lost the FM system. They didn't get it up and running until just about Christmas time. Jackson was having difficulty in computer lab and he is normally very good with computers. None of this was brought to my attention until many months into the school year. The teacher told me that Jackson wasn't focused or on task. He would be on a different website than everyone else. When I asked Jackson about this, he said that he couldn't hear her. I asked him, "Why? Isn't the teacher wearing the FM headset?" His answer was, "No."

Even with all of that, Jackson's grades didn't go down that low. We were working getting him to do his work more independently. I have had to work with him on his homework to keep his grades where they were and I was about ready to pass the fifth grade for the second time.

All of the stuff that we've done at *The Davis Center* has helped to keep him out of the resource center and from needing many accommodations. Although he is still struggling, and I can see his difficulties. When something goes too slow for him, he gets bored. When something goes too fast, he can't keep up with it. Seeing his frustration one evening, I decided to draw a bar graph. It contained his standings in spelling, reading, comprehending, math, word problems, paying attention and memory. For the most part, he is doing great across the board. He can get a hundred on a spelling test without even breaking a sweat. He can read with ease. His computation skills are great and he has an excellent memory. At times he has some trouble with comprehending, word problems and paying attention. When I see Jackson get frustrated, I just remind him about the bar graph. He can see where he needs work and where his strengths are. It helps him stay focused on what he needs to improve. Paying attention is an exercise that he can improve on if he focuses. His issues with comprehension and doing word problems are going to take a little more work, but it's easy to convince Jackson that he can do it when we take into account how far he has already come.

STORY RESPONSE

Jackson's mother is a caring mom who wants her son helped. She devotes many hours a day to making sure her son will succeed. Although she gets frustrated at times, her strength continues to rise above her frustrations to help him. I remember supporting her through many difficult periods of frustration. "What can I do to help my son?"

I wanted Stacey's story in this book because it exemplifies the frustrations of many parents. My *Davis Center* staff frequently supports the parents as well as the child making change. The changes we make can be life altering. Parents may need to change how they parent simply because the child is able to understand and communicate better. Sometimes this is harder for the parent than the child. As with Jackson, once one issue was resolved such as the hypersensitivity to sound, then other issues were more easily seen, such as the reading issues, and then these new skill deficits needed to be addressed. The road to success can be long for some people.

It is also not uncommon for children who have been diagnosed with processing problems early on, to do well with structured learning responses. The first Speech Pathologist provided him with skills that allowed him to succeed at that time. Obviously Jackson's intelligence provided him ways to function more appropriately with his new skills. However, his processing issues were still present. They simply were being demonstrated in different ways. Jackson became frustrated and the school personnel were puzzled. Something was missing for Jackson.

The changes obtained with The Listening Program were not unexpected. However, understanding my "Tree" analogy is important. The Listening Program is at the upper *Trunk* and/or the lower *Leaves and Branches*. One can make change with this program but the changes are often not the core foundational changes that make the most change and are not retained. This is why Jackson's mother reported that "Obviously, The Listening Program hadn't worked all that well" one year after it was finished and he had reverted back to having difficulties. His body had not been able to maintain the initial advances, because it had not been properly prepared.

I have found that I can make the most change for children the earlier that I have a chance to work with them. The brain is more malleable at earlier ages. It would have been better for Jackson to have received sound therapy interventions at the first indication of problems as a preschooler. He may have needed other therapies later in his development, but perhaps not as many. Because of the importance of developing sound processing skills in young children, I feel it's very important to start helping children with any form of developmental issue with sound therapy before moving into other supportive therapies.

Jackson's initial *DETP* had suggested AIT, Tomatis, and BioAcoustics. Jackson started AIT and immediately his decreased hearing hypersensitivities allowed him to feel more comfortable with his body and the world around it. One reason that he was able to respond to things better is because he no longer had to overreact to the sounds around him and he could tune into something like the radio. He was also less frustrated because he wasn't on sensory overload as much and his body had time to respond more appropriately.

He moved quickly into Tomatis and he became even more aware of his environment. Things began to fall into place for him more easily, yet he continued to have reading issues. His attention improved and he was able to focus better on what needed to be accomplished.

As I have previously mentioned, there is a big difference between AIT and Tomatis. *Sound Bodies through Sound Therapy* explains the differences in great detail. Jackson's mother mentioned the difference of the activities allowed during the sessions. While doing AIT, it is important to not stimulate the other senses in order to maximize the hearing sense. It is also important not to eat or drink during the sessions because this counteracts the impulse being stimulated with the AIT machine in use. So while doing AIT, it is best to sit quietly and listen. For some children, this of course, is very difficult so only simple, non-stimulating activities should be allowed such as the use of small manipulatives.

For Tomatis it is helpful to incorporate all of the senses, because the method is working on total development. One of the reasons that I prefer to emphasize a "total person" approach versus a sensory integration approach is because when only one issue is challenged to make change, it is that issue that is clearly addressed. However, the body wants to make change in many areas and be able to integrate all of the senses and skills, so I prefer to let the body direct the way it wants to make change and then have my staff support and challenge that direction versus having my staff directing the body to make change in only certain areas. It is a more natural progression of development.

Our *Read-Spell-Comprehend* program helps people with issues at the top of the *Leaves and Branches* of *The Tree* analogy. Jackson had progressed to this level after getting his needed foundational supportive change. He was able to use these skills to get through fourth grade, because the foundation was in place. However, he also began to integrate the skills he was learning with the Fast ForWord series more easily, again because the foundation was in place.

Jackson still has auditory processing issues. The FM system was suggested to support him with hearing his teachers more directly and with an intensity level just slightly louder than the surrounding background classroom noise. This system makes listening easier and more comfortable for him, allowing him to understand more of what he is learning and what is expected of him.

Jackson has made significant progress since first starting with me. However, his *DETP* also suggested BioAcoustics. Sometimes, it is this last piece, "The Maintenance of the Tree", that allows his body to make more progressive long term change. Perhaps this may support Jackson with even greater progress. Would Jackson also benefit from more Tomatis? Possibly, but this would only be determined from yearly Listening Test evaluations.

CHAPTER EIGHT

Trenton   PDD

"He would walk up to people and look them in the
eye. He started introducing himself to people.
He wanted to be known."

Turners Station, Kentucky: Karen glances across the table with a motherly look of understanding and compassion as she thoughtfully prepares to share her story.

Trenton was a happy little boy. We couldn't tell anything was wrong with him. When Trenton was seven-months old, he could say "Momma" and "Dadda." He had the normal jabber that babies do. At eight-months old, Trenton started having ear infections. He got a high fever and started crying and pulling on his ear. When we took him to the pediatrician, they gave him antibiotics. The antibiotics wouldn't work very well. They would work for a little while, but the ear infections would come back. He developed a pattern. He would get an ear infection in the fall and it would last until spring. This happened every year.

When he was about two-years old, he got his measles, mumps and rubella vaccine. Soon after he started to regress. He preferred to be alone and he wouldn't make eye contact. Trenton is the kind of kid who couldn't relax. He walked or moved nonstop, but he would do it in his room. He didn't want to be around anyone, and he became very quiet. He lost what words he had and wouldn't speak, he'd just grunt or cry. When he wanted something, he would either point to it or take me by the arm and show me. He would make a sound, but it wouldn't be a word. He was three-years old before he said his first words again. He learned to say, "bye-bye." That was the first thing he said after his regression.

It was at this time that we had Trenton evaluated for all the issues he was going through. He had to have ten characteristics to be categorized with autism. Trenton didn't have all ten. He had a few and that was enough to categorize him with the Pervasive Developmental Disorder. It has a very broad range, and could be considered severe to mild autism. It could be anything, and that's just a name they give your child when they can't categorize him any other way.

When Trenton turned four-years old, we had tubes put in his ears to take care of the ear infections he had been having all his life. His tonsils and adenoids were also removed. It helped a great deal. Trenton had less frequent ear infections, and didn't run the high fevers anymore.

When he was in kindergarten, the doctor put Trenton on a medicine called clonidine. That was for his aggressiveness because he couldn't relax and would just walk or constantly have to move. It was to help settle him down a little bit. Clonidine slowed him down tremendously. He was able to notice things more. He started making friends and he fit in more. He was actually able to sit and listen to a story being read. Trenton's autism wasn't very extreme. The only thing extreme was that he couldn't talk and he couldn't read.

Throughout Trenton's life, we put him in speech therapy. He was also prescribed the Secretin shot that is sometimes given to kids with autism. But because he was physically able to function, Trenton didn't need anything else. He was in special classes at school. Trenton did alright in school and he began to be more sociable. The teachers used a Pictures Exchange Card System where children communicate using pictures. We even tried an electronic talking board where Trenton could communicate by pushing buttons associated with words. We didn't use that for very long as

Trenton would play with it rather than use it in the correct manner.

Trenton has had the same pediatrician since he was two. His pediatrician never thought Trenton had autism. He just said Trenton was slow and that he would catch up with other kids his age. He has been in speech therapy for years. We never put him in anything else because there just isn't anything around that deals with autism where we live.

Trenton was getting older and he still wasn't where we thought he needed to be. He didn't like social gatherings. If we never left the house, he'd be just as happy. Trenton could catch on to things and learn if you demonstrated and did it first. He could ride a bike, but he could not talk to people or communicate with them. Trenton wouldn't even spend the night at his grandmother's house or anything, since he didn't like to go anywhere.

As Trenton got a little older, he became angry. He started hurting himself. When he was eight- or nine-years old, he would throw fits where he would hit his head or bite himself. His strength was unreal. I worked at the school and everyday as I would turn down the road to go to work, Trenton would start throwing a fit. He hated to go to school and would cry entering the building.

When we learned of another child who went to *The Davis Center*, his success story prompted me to look into it for Trenton. Trenton was eleven-years old when we first took him to *The Davis Center*. The *Diagnostic Evaluation for Therapy Protocol* was the first step we needed to take. Dorinne Davis told us that Trenton could be helped, and just needed two therapies. He needed Auditory Integration Training to be followed by Tomatis. We saw the print outs of his evaluations and we were willing to give it a try to do anything we could for Trenton. There isn't really anything out there and *The Davis Center* was a rare thing that we could do to help

Trenton.

During the AIT, Trenton did very well. He started to notice things more, and was more observant of the world. Before all this, Trenton had learned to repeat certain words. He just didn't use language on his own. If I tried to teach Trenton the word "dog," I would say "dog" and he would repeat it. He just wouldn't look at a dog and say, "dog." But now, Trenton would point to things and try to say them on his own. Things were clearer for him.

Because we come from Kentucky, we spent one whole month in New Jersey and put Trenton through all of his therapies at once. So we went straight into Tomatis after AIT and it's hard to tell at what time and from which therapy, but Trenton started to make certain changes. Trenton was sick the entire time because of the therapies and vomited every day. But when we finished his treatments and came home, Trenton was calmer. He quit vomiting and was happy to go back to school. He would walk up to people and look them in the eye. He started introducing himself to people. He wanted to be known. He said his first sentence while we were in New Jersey, "I want tea."

Since then, we've made three trips to New Jersey to put him through the 15-day Tomatis sessions. We're due back to put Trenton through an 8-day boost. It really has helped him a great deal. He started learning to read Dr. Seuss books and has gotten on track with reading. For the first time, he brings books for me to read to him and he can sit for awhile to listen. He has never done that before. Basically he has more understanding, and understands directions more clearly now. He can even name flash cards now.

Trenton has had some regressions that have happened in the past four months. But if we ask him, "Who's boy are you?" he can say, "Daddy's boy." We can even switch the question around and say, "Who's Daddy's boy?" and he'll say, "Trenton."

The teachers have seen a huge personality change. They were delighted to see Trenton so happy to be at school, and that his learning has improved. They have noted that he follows directions better and he can understand a two step verbal direction instead of just one. If you ask him to get the ball and bring it back, he can do both of those rather than just giving him one direction at a time.

Everyone has noticed the changes; he's even become closer to his brother. He tries to do everything that his brother does. He tries to say everything that his brother does. He never did that before. His brother could probably teach him more than anyone and now has the chance to do it.

STORY RESPONSE

My first impression of Trenton was that he appeared ordinary yet quiet. Once I introduced myself to him, I saw a young man with a beautiful smile struggling to figure out what was going on around him. The family–Mom, Dad, and an older brother had come to NJ to search for change for their son and brother. It was also apparent how very supportive they were.

Trenton's background is somewhat typical of many autistic children. His symptoms were on the autistic spectrum, yet he was labeled with the catchall, Pervasive Developmental Disorder (PDD) because autism is so broad based. His parents had sought help from different medical professionals to help them with his ear problems and aggressiveness. He received Speech Therapy, supported by the PECS system to support his language and communication skills. What *The Davis Center* did differently was to look at the whole child. Specifically, they determined a developmental protocol to make positive change, using the voice-ear-brain connection.

His parents related that I had suggested AIT and Tomatis, in that order. Because of distance and travel expenses, it is not uncommon for some clients to move directly from AIT into Tomatis. The two therapies work on totally different skills: AIT on the sense of hearing and Tomatis for listening or general sound processing. They do not necessarily require a break in between the two therapies. In fact, I encourage clients to move quickly into Tomatis (within six weeks of completion) so that the process of retraining the muscle started in AIT can be enhanced when Tomatis stabilizes the connection between both muscles in the middle ear.

With AIT, the stapedius muscle is retrained. It then allows sound to be vibrationally received by both the cochlea and vestibular system more accurately and clearly. With Tomatis, this process becomes stabilized because it massages and improves the interaction of the middle ear mechanisms for sound transmission.

During therapy, Trenton was ill for much of the time because of the impact on the vestibular system. It was being "balanced" so to speak. He was now receiving sound vibration in a different manner and his body was repatterning his responses to vibrational input. Motion sickness, vertigo, and the sensation of wanting to throw up are triggered from the vestibular portion of the ear. Trenton vomited daily because of the impact of the therapies on this portion of his ear. This response demonstrated where many of his initial imbalances were located. The body was trying to correct itself.

His learning skills began to increase because he was better able to tune in and learn about the world around him. He was able to understand more because he was better able to "take in" and receive information from his environment. He understood directions more clearly because he was better able to hear the sound differences in words and sentences, and therefore remember more of what he heard.

His parents also reported "regression" over the last four months of therapy. After a client leaves, the body needs time to integrate the changes and to stabilize itself. Some clients need more sessions in order to make sure the changes are retained. Some clients are able to move to a home program that utilizes the Tomatis concepts with special emphasis on the use of active voice work. By using Dr. Tomatis' concepts, it is the voice that becomes the body's stabilizer. The voice-ear-brain connection is stimulated by the Tomatis method; however, by training the voice to support and maintain the changes, the changes last longer and eventually become permanent. Dr. Tomatis' third law says that the improved listening over time results in permanently and unconsciously improving the voice-ear-brain connection. That is the path we are on with Trenton and all of our clients.

Many times, the parents of our clients speak about the changes they see, but say the school reports that they see no change as they may be looking for different types of change. For example, a child may not immediately make two grade level changes according to standardized testing, however, there is typically a change in their ability to take in and learn about the world around them. Other teachers report significant grade changes to the point that children frequently no longer need special education services. The fact that Trenton's teachers noticed the dramatic changes was very exciting as his changes were very significant. They began to see the child who was outwardly happy, but not able to share his happiness, become an aware and communicative child. He was now beginning to experience connections with others.

Because of the close warm, loving and mentoring relationship with his older brother, Trenton now experiments with "how it should be done". He now explores the many new opportunities to learn. His brother continues to be his role model helping him to explore new options.

CHAPTER NINE

Samuel   Autism

> "Instead of tuning people out, Samuel was joining
> and participating. He was starting to ask
> questions and putting sentences together."

Feasterville, Pennsylvania: Marie thinks for a minute trying to remember everything that has taken place over the last few years.

Samuel has just turned six, and it's been over four years that we have been noticing things about him. It was around 18-months when we realized he had issues. He wasn't talking and he wasn't responding to anything. His pediatrician ordered a hearing test. It was concluded that he could hear. He would turn his head toward sound, but in a room with a group of people, he would tune everyone out.

He liked to watch the Disney Channel, but different tones would make him cover his ears with his hands, and he'd start humming. When a child has autism, they normally develop "stimming" activities or activities that he can stimulate himself in some way. Samuel would move his hands back and forth. He used his index finger and his thumb to make a motion like a duck's beak quacking. He wouldn't make eye contact and he really didn't like to talk at all. Instead of asking for something like juice, he would take your hand and walk you over to the refrigerator. That was his way of showing us he wanted something.

We placed Samuel in an early intervention program. I called the Bucks County Association for Retarded Citizens or BARC. They referred me to the intermediate unit who set me up with the early intervention program. Samuel began getting speech therapy, occupational therapy and physical therapy. Therapists were sent from the Buck's County Intermediate Unit to come to the house. They stopped physical therapy when Samuel reached the age of three. Early intervention is normally from ages one to three and then the child goes into the preschool level.

Samuel went into a special needs classroom where they provided occupational therapy and speech in the classroom. When he was four, I decided to put him back in the autistic program. I had taken him out of it for a short period of time. His Applied Behavior Analysis program actually started at three and a half years old when I originally put him in the autistic program. During a Magnetic Resonance Imaging or MRI test, they found something about ventricular space in the head where spinal fluid is. In layman's terms, everything was normal but Samuel's head was rather big. Doctors mentioned that this placed Samuel on the high side just outside of normal. Now they are more commonly considering conditions such as Samuel's as a factor to look for in an infant as it may indicate early signs of autism.

While Samuel was in an autistic program, I also took him to a dietician. There was something different about my son's autism. He didn't have a problem with eating dairy products. He didn't test positive for any of the dairy allergies. Many kids can't break down those enzymes. They have digestive problems, allergies and rashes. Samuel never showed any of these signs.

I researched Auditory Integration Training and looked for places that I could take Samuel. I talked to some therapists and teachers. One speech therapist was against it saying she thought it would cause more harm than good. It is not a researched program and she knew of someone who had encountered adverse effects during AIT. The therapist really tried discouraging us. She also was saying that Samuel's sensitivities were getting worse, not better. I gave that careful consideration, but all the other input pointed toward AIT being something that would benefit Samuel. It was my decision to explore AIT further because Samuel is relatively intelligent. He is reading at age six. At the age of four, he knew his alphabet, colors and numbers. I continued looking at AIT.

The only thing close enough was *The Davis Center*. It was only two hours away. I looked at the website, and I got a few references. I called *The Davis Center* and they referred me to people who had gone through the programs and came out successfully. I was sufficiently impressed and called for an appointment.

The *Diagnostic Evaluation for Therapy Protocol* was somewhat shocking at first because it was rather hard to understand, but Dorinne explained it. The Listening Test indicated that Samuel was sensitive to sound. The two lines on the Listening Test are the way sound enters his ears and he processes it. The closer the lines are, the better his listening abilities are. His initial testing showed that his lines were very far apart. When Dorinne explained everything, she made it all come together. It makes a lot of sense the way everything is processed. Your ears are closest to the brain. Samuel wasn't responding very well to his environment. I now understood why, and was ready to help develop those skills any way I could.

AIT was rough. We had to make a two hour drive to get there, and we had to stay between the two 30-minute sessions scheduled three and one half hours apart. There wasn't much to do to spend those three hours in between. We would go to lunch or go shopping just to find something to do. However it was worth it when teachers actually saw dramatic change after his first session.

Samuel didn't like the headphones at first. He didn't want anything on his ears. I gave him credit cards to play with as an incentive to put the headphones on and it worked rather well. He started putting the headphones on with little trouble. During AIT, they just put him in a small room and he has to sit there the entire time. It was hard for him to sit still, but we worked through it.

The immediate results were very encouraging. He started using language more and responded better. He started turning toward the person talking and listening to what they were saying. He was so much more interactive during the first month. Instead of tuning people out, Samuel was joining and participating. He was starting to ask questions and putting sentences together.

We went directly into the 15-day Tomatis, and basically stayed in New Jersey for the whole month of November. Tomatis was so much easier because Samuel could do things. He could move around if he wanted, and there were different things to do like read or jump on the trampoline. If he wanted to doze off because he was tired, that was fine as long as he kept his headphones on the entire time.

Samuel was doing much better after Tomatis. He was listening and talking more. He normally didn't talk on the phone, but he was getting more comfortable with that. He would talk to his father while we were away in New Jersey and they would have decent conversations. He was also better at answering questions.

We took time off in December and then did another session of Tomatis in January. When Samuel went back to school, the teachers were really blown away by his improvement. He was very attentive in class and was following directions very well. The teachers noted that he was calmer and since his hearing sensitivities had gone away, he was responding better in class.

To explain it a little better, Dorinne focused on his hypersensitive hearing. Dorinne desensitized his hearing, and sounds weren't agitating his ears as much. During the Tomatis session, they have one or two sessions where they gave him a microphone. We had to get him to talk into it by having him read a book, so he could hear his own voice. That helped him to realize what his own voice was and how to use it more.

It just seems that he keeps making progress on a steady basis. His hearing is better, his speech is coming along, and Samuel just seems to be dealing better overall in his environment. Now we are doing 8-day boosts. We will be doing another during his spring break. Everything Dorinne has suggested has worked tremendously, and we're just going along with the program. If she suggests doing something, we don't hesitate to put Samuel through it. The lines that I spoke of earlier are almost together like they should be. He has a couple dips up and down. That's why we are taking him back to *The Davis Center* to have those ironed out, as we think he can benefit from it again.

STORY RESPONSE

Samuel looked like an adorable pixie when I first met him. His face was so expressive of fear and pain. He had large eyes that seemed to say to you, "I don't know if I can trust you because my world is so uncomfortable". He was all over the place exploring, yet afraid at the same time. My heart went out to him and I knew I could help him.

Most of my clients at *The Davis Center* have savvy parents willing to look for the best for their child and obtain it at whatever the cost or inconvenience. Although their Speech Pathologist had warned Samuel's parents against AIT, it was their persistence that brought him to our center. They happened to find me under the category of an AIT search. Little did they know at that time the extent of services we were able to offer Samuel.

Because of inconclusive studies, and those research studies measuring inappropriate outcomes, research in the United States has not been overly supportive of the AIT method. As such, many associations have suggested not using the method. However, as my research indicates in *Sound Bodies through Sound Therapy*, AIT works on retraining the acoustic reflex muscle and helps one type of hearing hypersensitivity. When appropriately indicated by testing, AIT is a very important part of one's therapy protocol. With an understanding of its use, its potential outcome is understood.

For those who have been warned or are worried about adverse effects, I suggest reading the chapter on AIT in *Sound Bodies through Sound Therapy*. It will help in understanding why AIT is an important step and one that is necessary for some children. AIT assists the repatterning of how the body processes certain sensory information. If the therapy protocol is adhered to, as indicated by the *DETP*, any adverse effects quickly become more appropriate responses. All too often, when only AIT is administered, the person gets stuck at a certain level and has difficulty moving beyond that level. The use of my "Tree" analogy is crucial to one's success.

As his mother indicated, Samuel began making positive change immediately with AIT. His *Hearing Sensitivity Audiogram* changed nicely. He then moved into the Tomatis method. It is this method that uses the Listening Test that Samuel's mother mentioned. The Listening Test is proprietary to the Tomatis method, from which the individualized programming is determined. It is based on the voice-ear-brain connection established by Dr. Alfred Tomatis and reflects all of the issues identified in the *Trunk* of *The Tree*. It provides information on listening and sound processing.

Samuel's attitude during all of the therapies was impressive. This fearful young boy knew almost immediately that he needed to make a change. He didn't like the headphones at first. He was fearful of anything different. After a few times, he appeared to instinctively know it was helping and accepted the discomfort in order to make change. He was truly courageous.

As a therapist, watching Samuel change was very rewarding. Yes, he began using more language, and yes, he was listening better, and yes, he was more interactive. But what was exciting for me, was to see the person inside of that fearful body beginning to emerge. Samuel was becoming more comfortable with who he was and he began to reach out to others. It was great to watch the fear subside.

Samuel still has a ways to go to grow and develop. He will need more of the Tomatis method and active use of his voice to establish better overall responses. Once his Listening Test indicates this, it will be possible for him to move into the *Leaves and Branches* level of *The Tree* analogy. Sometimes it is easy to determine from just the Listening Test what therapy should be suggested next. However, many clients also require the Advanced level–*Diagnostic Evaluation for Therapy Protocol* or *A-DETP*, because they need a higher level skill set evaluation in order to determine what comes next.

As Samuel grows older, the *Body Maintenance* level of *The Tree* analogy may also have to be revisited. His initial *DETP* did not suggest BioAcoustics, yet as he grows and develops, and as his body changes, it may be suggested at the *A-DETP* level.

Samuel has come a very long way in his development. Sound-based therapies have been instrumental in helping him respond better, learn more easily, and interact with others more appropriately. The sound therapies have helped him, as well as complementing all of his other therapies and learning processes.

CHAPTER TEN

Zachary

Autism, PDD, ADHD

> "He went from a kid that you couldn't understand to a
> kid that you could understand in just two weeks."

Ashland, Pennsylvania: Carrie's slight New England accent starts to come through as she recalls Zachary's first few years.

When Zachary was a child, he would cry and have tantrums. When he started to talk, he would just babble. I couldn't understand him at all; no one could. He was frustrated and I was frustrated. He was cutting off the beginnings and the endings of words. He was showing signs of aggression and he was always biting people. He would even bite me at times. He also used to chew things, like chew the end of his shoelaces right off his shoes. He would chew pencils and cardboard. He would chew things for so long and then spit them out. I would find little chewed up things all over the house.

When we took him for his three-year old check up, his pediatrician said that he was fine. He knew his numbers and the alphabet, however I knew he didn't quite know fifty words. His pediatrician also told me that he was a boy and boys are known for developing slower. The pediatrician wouldn't believe that I was noticing certain issues with my son. I just couldn't name them. I didn't feel like our pediatrician was helping much at all. Eventually, I ended up changing pediatricians.

I was home with Zachary most of the day and I just felt something was not right. There were so many things. He used to gag on different textures of food. He only liked crunchy things like Doritos or cereal that made noise in his mouth. Plus he only liked certain kinds of clothes, like his pajamas which were comfortable for him.

When he started school, he would come home and want to change immediately. He would live in his pajamas if I let him. Now, he doesn't mind as much, but it was pretty bad back then. He also wouldn't acknowledge things going on around him if he was focused on something else. I could yell his name behind his back, but he wouldn't turn around to look at me if he was interested in something else.

A few months after Zachary's 3-year old check up, I called an early intervention program. I wanted them to help him with his language. They brought everybody to meet him including an occupational therapist, a physical therapist and a speech therapist. It was from this early intervention program that I accidentally learned Zachary was autistic. The therapists said that Zachary needed to be desensitized to certain textures that touch his skin or go in his mouth. When I heard that, I thought to myself that I had heard that somewhere before. Maybe I had seen a show or something and it rang a bell with me. Zachary's therapists told me that they were not doctors, so they could only give me recommendations. They wrote up a report and came back to me with everything Zachary was qualified to get. They noted that Zachary might have a Pervasive Developmental Disorder and Attention Deficit Hyperactive Disorder.

The therapists suggested a hearing test. I called the pediatrician and he gave me a hard time, as he didn't want to do it. I told him that all I asked for was a hearing test. I mentioned that if Zachary had a hearing difficulty, we should fix it. While he was fighting me, that's when I decided to change pediatricians. Zachary was about three and a half years old at the time.

One day I was watching a morning show on television and they did a story on Tomatis. The story mentioned that people with

ADHD, autism and all sorts of other issues could benefit from Tomatis therapy. So I looked it up on the computer. I found *The Davis Center* and looked into it. When I called, I set up an appointment and took Zachary to get evaluated.

After the *Diagnostic Evaluation for Therapy Protocol*, Dorinne explained the next steps we needed to take. I decided to go ahead as Dorinne recommended and start with Tomatis. I didn't want to go through life wondering if I hadn't have tried it, would it have helped Zachary? I thought the best thing to do was give it a try and then I wouldn't have to go through life wondering. We set a schedule and went to New Jersey in August for fifteen days.

We put him through Tomatis and we saw changes all over the place. He stopped biting and his speech became better. When we returned home after the first session, the early intervention team came to the house and they couldn't believe it. They could understand what he was saying. After Zachary adjusted to the Tomatis, he was so much clearer that everyone commented on it. The therapists were all looking at each other in wonder at how drastically he had changed. He went from a kid that you couldn't understand to a kid that you could understand in just two weeks. Some people get more out of Tomatis than others and Zachary really benefited from it.

We went through a second session of Tomatis and he was doing even better. He started reading books. He actually had a few audio-books that he memorized. When I would read the book to him, he could pick out when I mispronounced a word or if I skipped one. I thought that was remarkable because not only was he memorizing speech, he was also able to identify where words belonged in the book.

One of the phenomenal things about Dorinne is that she

gives us instructions for when we go home. She tells me things that I can expect to notice. She told me that Zachary should listen to Mozart in the morning and Gregorian Chants in the evening. When I read to him, I was supposed to read into his right ear. So, we did those things and it helped. He responded better when I read into his right ear. But that's not all, there were other things she told me to keep an eye out for and they all happened.

Dorinne told me some things about his writing abilities. She told me that he would start writing more and that he would do it on his own. Before Zachary never liked to write at all, although he does now more than he ever has. He is getting more confident in himself. That's how Tomatis has helped him with his self-esteem.

This is why I find it so interesting. Dorinne shows me from her graphs that there are things I need to look for when I get home. It all depends on where Zachary is in therapy, but we're looking for different things at different times. When his listening levels change, Dorinne can pick up on the other changes that are going to take place. When I mentioned that he didn't like to write, she told me that she could see that from the graph. I thought it was interesting that Dorinne can read a person from the graphs she makes. I feel really comfortable with her because she knows what she is doing. When I'm not comfortable with someone, I'll switch to someone else, as I did with my pediatrician. I'm glad to take Zachary back to *The Davis Center*; he won't be changing therapists this time. Dorinne does a wonderful job at explaining things and telling me what to notice.

He is in kindergarten now because his birthday is at the end of August. I had been able to keep Zachary in the early intervention program for an extra year. We didn't put him in school until he was six. Because of Zachary's classification of autism, PDD and ADHD, the school wrote up an IEP for him. When they were writing up his goals, I told the teachers that if they had trouble communicating to Zachary that it might help to talk into his right ear. When they agreed to do that, I felt like Zachary was going to do just fine in school.

Zachary wasn't finished with his therapies yet. After the third session of Tomatis, Zachary became a little more sociable. He tried to initiate conversations and make friends. Teachers noticed that he was friendlier and he was trying to make connections with other kids, something he had never done before.

When we returned from the next 8-day Tomatis boost, we observed how Zachary started noticing things around him. He could be distracted by them even if he was focused on something else. When a neighbor was mowing his grass one day, I opened the door to make it cooler in the house. It was a nice day and I wanted to let in the sun. Zachary asked me to close the door because he couldn't concentrate over the sound of the lawn mower. This was a huge change because I remember yelling his name behind his back and he wouldn't respond when he was focused on something. Now he was responding, and he was able to take in more of the world around him.

We are very willing to keep up the therapies because we have seen such a difference. Some of the other people you meet there are great to talk to as well. We've talked to so many people whose lives have been changed by the therapies at *The Davis Center*. It was neat to hear their stories and see how they had benefited from it. It's a nice little support group too knowing that other people have gone through the same things. Now I get asked for my opinion, instead of the other way around when I was asking other people for their opinions.

Zachary was pretty young and I think we just hit it at the right time. I really didn't have time to try anything else with him. I guess I am fortunate that I chose to try *The Davis Center* first. I don't think that he would be doing as well as he is if it hadn't been for *The Davis Center*. He wouldn't be as far as he is now.

I know that it has helped greatly with Zachary's schooling. He is in class with the other kids all day long except for speech every Friday for a half an hour every week. He used to have occupational therapy every week, but they cut that back to every other week. He doesn't like getting taken out of class. He still needs a little extra help to some extent. He still doesn't like some of the paint textures when he is in art class, but he tolerates it. He colors more than he ever did, as the crayons don't annoy him as much. I think that's more of a writing thing because it's a little hard for him to stay in the lines and control his hand movements. I'm not very sure whether he likes to color or not, but he is tolerating it.

STORY RESPONSE

Zachary was the cutest little boy when I first met him, his round face and impish eyes belied the fact that he was lost within himself. Although I appreciate his mother's accolades, the entire staff at *The Davis Center* helps accomplish the "miracles" we achieve. It is the *DETP* which sets us on the right path, and then my dedicated staff supports the person on their therapy pathway. We are a team! Watching Zachary blossom was exciting for us. His parents were supportive at every stage of his development.

Zachary's *DETP* indicated the need for Tomatis as the starting place. He did not have the type of hearing hypersensitivity that would have required AIT. However, he did have hypersensitivity to sound through his bone conduction listening responses. These responses told me that he was unable to connect to the world outside of his body unless he was pulled out, for example, by calling his name to get his direct attention. This response to the world limited Zachary in his ability to learn language and communication skills.

When Zachary began his Tomatis method listening program, he made very quick and positive changes. The Tomatis method addresses and modifies many sensory integration imbalances. Zachary displayed many of these imbalances by: gagging on certain food textures, only liking crunchy foods, not liking certain clothing textures, blocking out sounds around him, and liking to put things in his mouth to chew. These issues all have a connection to the semi-circular canals and vestibule in the inner ear. By correcting how sound and vibration stimulate this portion of the ear, many of the issues resolve themselves. Some children also benefit from the ancillary effects of the indirect branching of the cranial nerves passing through this portion of the ear; again with the outcome that the issues resolve themselves.

The overall effect of all sound therapies is to allow the body to regain its natural form and function. The voice-ear-brain connection, whether from the inside of the body outward, as with Tomatis, or the outside of the body inward, as with BioAcoustics, supports this *Cycle of Sound*. Once Zachary began the Tomatis method, his body found ways to balance itself, allowing his sensory system to respond more appropriately—eliminating the gagging on certain food textures, allowing for more food variety, enjoying more than pajamas as clothes, tuning into the sound world around him, and decreasing his need to chew on things. Zachary was finally able to learn about what was happening outside of his body and he quickly learned to tune into that information for better overall development.

Eventually Zachary's Listening Test, will reach good levels and indicate that Zachary can stop returning for treatment sessions. When he reaches puberty, however, he may benefit from additional sessions. Many children, especially boys, can benefit from additional sessions of Tomatis and for some AIT while experiencing the hormonal changes brought on by puberty. While an adolescent body is changing, the changes often bring about imbalances. Many parents have discovered the value of helping their children "over the hump" by having them do additional sessions of Tomatis during these years, to help prepare them for adulthood. Self-esteem and self-worth are inherently established once a person can processes incoming information appropriately.

CHAPTER ELEVEN

Amy

Speech & Language Issues
Central Auditory Processing Disorder

> "She was able to retain new words that she was learning.
> She was able to spell them correctly when she was
> asked to recall them. She reads very fluidly now whereas
> her reading had been choppy and one word at a time before."

Ridgewood, NJ: Diane had just washed the dishes as she sat down to talk about Amy.

*A*my was diagnosed through school with speech and language development issues, although it was noted that it was related to auditory processing. There wasn't any formal medical diagnosis; it was done through school while in the third grade.

Amy had been a fairly normal child from birth. She did cry a great deal, but that's considered colic. Other than that, she seemed fine even though she did experience some developmental delays. She was a preemie twin born seven weeks prematurely. Brendan, her twin, was also developmentally delayed, but doctors said that was common with kids who were born early. Brendan turned out fine. Even though my daughter's developmental delays are only slight, she did experience some things that caused us to notice that she had issues.

Amy had a slight hearing sensitivity. She could hear airplanes and fire trucks much sooner than any of us could. But they didn't seem to bother her or anything. It wasn't as if her hearing was so sensitive that the sounds annoyed her or hurt her ears. While she could hear things were noticeable. When we told her something or asked her very well, she did experience issues with her hearing that were noticeable. When we told her something or asked her do a chore, she would just look at us as if she didn't understand what we were saying. Knowing that she was able to hear, this response, we learned, was part of her inability to process information.

Amy also never knew how to wind down to go to sleep. She was always worried about one thing after another and it would keep her up at night. She constantly came down the steps at night to talk or to ask me about these things. She wondered if she had done something wrong or if she had hurt someone's feelings as she replayed her day in her mind while trying to go to sleep. These were things that shouldn't have bothered her, but they did.

When Amy was in the second grade, her spelling wasn't good at all and her reading was very slow. When she would sound out a word on one page, she wouldn't know it when she saw it again on another page. If a child is struggling in class, the school will ask the parents if they want the child tested. So, I agreed to have Amy tested because I had been asking all along why Amy wasn't doing so well. In the report from the school, it stated that there was a discrepancy in Amy's auditory processing. The reason they stated her issue that way was because she has a high IQ, but she can't present it well. She can verbally present what she knows, but she can't write what she knows. She might be able to do it one day, but she forgets the next. So the school started to give her extra help. She was still in her regular class, but they had a support class that she would visit in the morning four days a week for half an hour.

Amy's schoolwork was getting a little better. They reviewed her work everyday and went over everything with her. The repetition helped a little, but it didn't help her retain information for long term use. It didn't help her improve her reading or spelling.

On a recommendation from a friend, we tried the Feingold diet. It eliminates anything artificial in her diet. It is also known as the ADHD diet, a diet for individuals with Attention Deficit Hyperactivity Disorder, and can help with learning and processing issues. We thought it couldn't hurt, so we decided to try it. It helped a little, and she was able to stay focused a little better. I started to think that she might have ADD or ADHD. However the testing at the school ruled out ADD as a possibility. I guess some kids can have some of the issues and not be ADD or ADHD.

Through a friend of mine whose daughter has Williams syndrome, we were told about *The Davis Center*. So we made the appointment to go for the initial evaluation and the *Diagnostic Evaluation for Therapy Protocol*. After the evaluation, it was suggested that she do the Tomatis therapy. Dorinne's diagnosis was that Amy had abnormal auditory perception that was unspecified. Amy's hearing threshold levels indicated normal hearing except in the right ear which demonstrated borderline hearing levels. Even though Amy had no indicators for sensitive hearing, she did have borderline hearing levels that meant her hearing was slightly below where it should be. Amy began the Tomatis program between fourth and fifth grade.

Doing Tomatis was great. That's what finally helped in a big way. Her sleepless nights went away. That was one of the first things that changed after the Tomatis. She wasn't bothered by everything anymore. The temper tantrums she
would have all the time, also eased up after Tomatis. These things all seemed normal to me. It was just a child being worried like a little worry wart or having a temper tantrum like someone who didn't get her way. Little did I know that it could all be connected to a slight hearing abnormality that was now being treated.

I put her through Tomatis between fourth and fifth grade because the sixth grade is the beginning of middle school. If she was classified, the school would not allow her to take a foreign language. Classified children are put into a resource support class because the school thinks a foreign language will overwhelm them. Amy didn't want that. This was motivation for doing the Tomatis method.

During fifth grade, her grades came up immensely. She was reading better. She was more focused on her work. She was able to retain new words that she was learning. She was able to spell them correctly when she was asked to recall them. She reads very fluently now whereas her reading had been choppy and one word at a time before.

When she entered the sixth grade, they mainstreamed her. She wasn't classified for a resource support class and she was able to take a foreign language. That's the main thing that *The Davis Center* did for Amy. She doesn't have to go through life getting held back because she can't present her true IQ. Teachers feel she will no longer be overwhelmed, and look forward to challenging her.

STORY RESPONSE

Amy was the kind of young lady who would have been able to "make it" without assistance. However, her inner self and true intelligence would never have been seen by others. There are many Amy's in the world today. They "make it" without assistance. They also begin to question themselves as they get older. They wonder why others around them can do things so easily while they struggle. This is also questioned because they know that they are smarter than the others who appear to accomplish things easily. "What's wrong with me?" they might ask their parents. Parents may lovingly saying, "Nothing, you just learn differently than they do. You know how smart you are! Look at how well you do." Of course, the child will question that response yet unconsciously work at believing it because their inner self knows it's true. However, life would be easier if the body was better balanced and that is how sound therapy helps. The body is brought into balance.

What happened in Amy's case is that she was able to have that inner self come out because the incoming information now made more sense to her body. She was able to process all sound stimulation more effectively, thereby making more sense of speech, language, words, inflections, rhythms, intonations, and so much more that is associated with language. Once the language was better understood, her reading skills fell into place as well. Reading is both a visual and an auditory process. Although the visual must be in place to see the combinations of letters and words on a page, it is the auditory letter sound and word combinations that make up sentences necessary for language compre-hension that allow the reader to comprehend the printed word better.

Amy did have some early indicators as a baby for possible developmental issues. Early indicators of future issues can be things like fussiness as a baby, eating challenges, enjoying excessive sensory input like spinning or rocking, overreaction to sounds, underreacting to sounds, a clinging to mom, wanting (or not wanting) to be held, moving from sitting to walking without crawling, excessive gagging or reflux, and/or delay in speech and language skills. It behooves parents and physicians to be aware of these possibilities and seek help for their children or patients at the earliest possible age. It is the voice-ear-brain connection, discovered by Dr. Tomatis and further refined by my Davis Addendum to the Tomatis Effect that is necessary for a sound foundation for stable development. The earlier this connection is fully established the better. The brain is malleable during the developmental years. The idea that the earlier that brain change occurs, the more the brain can adapt to change overall has been validated by numerous brain researchers.

At the end of Amy's therapy regimen, I could see how much better she felt about herself. It showed in her body's posture and stance, as well as how she responded to new challenges. As her mother says, "her intelligence now has time to be presented."

CHAPTER TWELVE

Taylor

ADHD, OCD
Dsylexia, Tourette's Syndrome

> "He had to listen to the sounds twice a day for eleven minutes. The tics almost immediately subsided."

Wayne, Pennsylvania: Jennifer commands the dogs to get quiet as a neighbor knocks on the back door. "I'm sorry. I'm in the middle of something," she whispers softly to her neighbor, "I'll call you."

Taylor had a very hard time maintaining friendships. It was a culmination of things about Taylor that he just couldn't help. When he first started going to school, he had plenty of friends. He started developing some behaviors that caused the other kids to distance themselves. He would interrupt a conversation and say something that just didn't coincide with it. There might be a few kids talking about football and he would interrupt with, "Did you know that ants can carry up to ten times their weight?" He also had a thing about invading space. Instead of walking with you, he would walk in front of you and almost on top of you. He wasn't the kind to get his face too close to yours, but he would invade your space with his body. That was annoying for kids as well.

We took Taylor to a behaviorist to see if there was anything that could be done to help him. Actually we took him to see many doctors throughout his life starting when he was in the second grade. Although this particular behaviorist we took him to see didn't believe in giving Taylor medications, which I thought was a very good thing. This behaviorist believed in cognitive behavioral therapy. He worked with Taylor and taught him how to deal with his anxieties. The behaviorist also told us that Taylor had some disabilities, Obsessive-Compulsive Disorder or OCD compounded with Attention Deficit Disorder. That explained a few things to me.

Since OCD is anxiety driven, Taylor had a hard time coping in school. It became increasingly difficult when the other kids started to pick on him about his behaviors. He started to develop tics and his head would start shaking. He loved playing soccer and as he loved running up and down the field. The other kids would notice his head shaking, and they'd point and laugh, which would make it worse. Every behavior he started to develop would get worse as the kids kept picking on him about them. He won't eat off of the same fork or drink out of the same cup someone else has touched. So kids would intentionally touch his fork. That was one of the things. There was another. One of the twitches he had was in his eye. He would blink his eye, which made him look like he was winking at you. Kids would say, "Quit winking at me." This obviously made it blink worse. The anxiety in him would cause his twitches to increase and it just escalated the entire situation. The more he did it, the more he got teased. The more he got teased, the more he did it. A cruel cycle, which seemed to have no end.

To compound the problems with Taylor, he struggled with dyslexia. By the time he was in the third grade, we knew he had more than just a basic reading problem. We lived in Maryland at the time and Taylor attended a Catholic school. They aren't really prepared to deal with special needs students with reading or behavioral problems. They just don't have the funding.

It was about this time that we decided to move from Maryland to Pennsylvania. We had two thoughts concerning Taylor and his schooling once we made this change. First, we thought to put him in a public school where there might be better funding to deal with his particular needs. Second, we thought it might benefit Taylor if we put him back a year. Taylor had always been one of the youngest kids in his class because his birthday fell in June, at the end of the school year. By the time his birthday came around, most of the kids in his class were almost a year older than he was. We thought if we kept him in the third grade for the next school year, that he would be among kids more his age.

At the public school, they ran plenty of tests on Taylor. They wouldn't give him a label because that would be politically incorrect. They did however say that he had an issue with reading and short term memory. We took it from there. We took Taylor to a specialist who was involved in the Wilson Approach. The specialist hit the nail on the head and diagnosed Taylor with dyslexia. The Wilson Approach is a two-way approach that incorporates the Wilson Reading System® with Fast ForWord. The Wilson Reading System is a multisensory structured language program that helps a student master reading, starting with the smallest unit of sound and progressing through fluent word recognition and even working with students at a higher level of cognition known as metacognition or thinking about thinking. Fast ForWord is a computer-based interactive training program that takes a student through a series of exercises and automatically adjusts to the student's increasing level of competence. Taylor worked with the specialist all summer long on the Wilson approach.

When Taylor went on to middle school, teachers gave him an Individualized Education Plan. They gave him a learning support teacher. He goes to her room twice a week and he can go whenever he has any free time. If he needs to review for a test, he can go and get extra help from her. He's also had the same counselor, Andy, for a few years and he has really begun to know Taylor. Andy keeps a good eye on him. He will call Taylor down to the office and talk to him. If he sees something happen at lunch or in the halls, Andy will ask Taylor what it was about. Andy will enlighten him on invading space or interrupting a conversation. Andy just doesn't talk to Taylor about it. He shows him how it feels. Andy will get real close to him and ask Taylor how that feels. Taylor will respond with, "Uncomfortable." Although, Andy knows Taylor understands.

The kids who were picking on Taylor in the new school really took it to another level. It just wasn't saying things to him or touching his fork at lunch anymore. A few of the kids created a website called, "Kill Taylor." It seems that many of the students were accessing it from the library right there in the school. Taylor knew all about it. One day Taylor mentioned something to a friend of his. It made us all very uneasy. "My life is very sad. I don't want to live anymore."

Our son's friend told his mother, and she came to us out of concern. We took him to a therapist. The therapist never really thought he would actually take his own life. But an alarm had gone off for all of us and we had to figure out what we could do to help him. My sister had mentioned Tomatis to us before. We didn't know what that could do for a child who has expressed not wanting to live anymore.

Dorinne had attended my sister's wedding. My sister mentioned my son to Dorinne and she agreed to see Taylor. Dorinne suggested that we talk to her before doing anything else. She wanted to see what she could do for him first. It just so happened that we had set an appointment for a neurologist, but we couldn't get Taylor into see him for months. We ended up seeing Dorinne first anyway. The neurologist might have prescribed medications, but that didn't happen.

After Dorinne conducted the *Diagnostic Evaluation for Therapy Protocol* on Taylor, I noticed several things that were remarkable. Dorinne asked me if anyone had ever mentioned Tourette's syndrome to me. She also asked, "Did you ever notice that when Taylor speaks he clears his throat?" I said I hadn't noticed. Actually, I had noticed it a little, but I thought it was from his OCD. It never crossed my mind that it could be something else. Dorinne pointed out that clearing his throat could be an indication of Tourette's. Then Dorinne mentioned something else. Dorinne was showing us his test results and describing things that were right on the money. She pointed out that there was a period between third grade to about fifth grade where something happened. She didn't know exactly what it was. When I thought about this timeframe, I realized that it was the time in his life when we had moved from Maryland. That was a monumental time in his life. It was a disturbing time for him. I thought, "How could she know that." My husband and I looked at each other and said, "There's something to this."

I've heard of people with dyslexia who also have Tourette's and I'm not sure why the two go hand in hand. I'm really not sure if they do go hand in hand or if it's just more common than not. My child was in real need of specialized treatment. Tourette's, dyslexia, OCD and ADD to name only the few we knew up to this point. It was time to let Dorinne do her thing and see what she could do for him. We took Taylor to the neurologist anyway since we had already scheduled the appointment and it doesn't hurt to have several opinions from various resources. The neurologist confirmed what Dorinne had told us about Taylor having Tourette's. That locked it down for me.

Taylor was thirteen and at the end of the seventh grade when we put him through the Auditory Integration Training which lasted ten days. We went to Cherry Hill, New Jersey which was only a forty-five minute drive from where we live. AIT had been offered there as an outreach. Dorinne came down twice during the AIT for testing, but there is a sound therapist there the rest of the time who is certified in everything. After the first five days, Dorinne came down to test all the kids to see if the program needs to be adjusted. We went to her office in Budd Lake for the final results.

Taylor had an unbelievable response to AIT. It was an adventure for him. He didn't have to go to school. We went to AIT in the morning for thirty minutes, but Taylor didn't have to go back to school. It didn't make sense to leave Cherry Hill since we had to come back a few hours later for another thirty minutes. We stayed in Cherry Hill and found things to do. He loved the "Mom and Taylor" time we spent between listening sessions. I remember bringing my daughter Lauren one day. She just wanted to see what was happening. Taylor had a bad day that day, as the focus wasn't just on him. That was just one bad day though. It was the first time in years that I felt that connected with him. He was really benefiting from AIT and I saw changes immediately.

One day while in Cherry Hill, we went to buy shoes for Taylor. When we went to the store, Taylor opened the door for me and let me walk in ahead of him. I always had to remind Taylor to watch that the door didn't swing back and hit someone walking in behind us. But not this time. I turned back and he was holding the door open for me. He didn't normally do that either because he would try to practically walk on top of you.

During AIT, some changes occurred that were just remarkable. Taylor has always been a rather kind person. That's one thing people always said about him. But he was even more kind to people. He also started to properly enunciate his words rather than mumble at an inaudible level.

One astonishing thing I never expected to happen, really made a lasting impression.

The staff at *The Davis Center* had told me that Taylor could experience physical growth. It was an interesting thing they were telling me and I had no idea how correctly they had made that call. Taylor had always been so thin and small. I always thought he was just a late bloomer. My husband and I are average height and our doctor told us that Taylor was going to be about average when he decided to start growing. This year in his physical, he had jumped up in height and weight. It was a tremendous growth spurt which continued every couple of months. I have to constantly buy him a new pair of shoes. It's like his feet are growing by the day and the rest of his body is drastically trying to catch them. Not only is it due to his reaching puberty, but the huge changes taking place in him because of the therapies. It affects the entire body and causes so many things to correct themselves. I was astounded. I never thought that such changes would occur due to sound-based therapies. Just the simple act of listening to music could cause all this to happen to my son, when the doctor said it would never happen.

After AIT, we gave him a break for a weekend and went right into Tomatis. It was his fourteenth birthday over the weekend, so we celebrated. Then on Monday, we were on our way to *The Davis Center*. It was about two hours away. So we decided to stay in a hotel. My dad lived close by and he would come to take Taylor out on his boat or we would have lunch with him. When we started making the drive, Taylor thought the drive was a drag, although he was excited about Tomatis, and made preparations for the trip. He would put bottles of water in the car and bring snacks like fruits and things.

During the first session of Tomatis, I had to read for forty-five minutes and I had to keep my voice very animated. It is like reading a story to a child and you have to keep the child interested. Taylor may not have liked the drive because it took a lot out of him, but he loved the therapy. He liked how it made him feel, and he believed it was helping him. He told Dorinne one day, "My mind feels a lot clearer. Not so foggy." His personality was changing. He became much more aware of his boundaries. He was no longer trying to invade a person's space and his social skills were getting better. His statements were more relevant to the conversation and he was no longer interrupting.

When we finished the first session of Tomatis, we took a 30-day break. Then we returned again for fifteen days. We then took a two-month break and did the 8-day boost at Cherry Hill. When Dorinne visited at Cherry Hill, she was concerned about Taylor's twitching. She was concerned that when he returned to school after the summer, his twitching might put him back to where he was before he began therapy if kids started picking on him again. So at the end of the 8-day boost, we started BioAcoustics. She asked us to come to *The Davis Center* and do a voiceprint. He had to speak for forty-four seconds and then a graph was created. A week later, we went up and met with the lady who does the BioAcoustics. She had analyzed his voiceprint. She focused in on the area that was creating the tics. They created special sounds for Taylor that were based on the specific frequencies Taylor had out of balance. He had to listen to the sounds twice a day for eleven minutes. The tics almost immediately subsided.

Then two and a half months into it, he stopped listening to the sounds. It became a battle to get him to do it. The tics were coming back. I didn't know what to do. The next time we saw Dorinne, she asked Taylor how he was doing with the BioAcoustics. I told her that it was hard to even get him to do it. She thought for a second and then mentioned that he was going through puberty and that he can change quickly. BioAcoustics deals with the energy of a person and any changes that take place within a person's body will change the voiceprint. The sounds that were programmed earlier were no longer good for Taylor. His body could no longer tolerate the sounds that were originally prescribed. Taylor needed to do another voiceprint. Because Taylor was going through puberty, they had to do a new voiceprint every three months. After they did another voiceprint, Taylor went back to listening with no problem. Everything gets readjusted and just puts his world on an even keel.

My husband thought since all this had helped Taylor so much, that he wanted to do BioAcoustics for himself. He had started experiencing some signs of aging and he thought maybe it could help. When they evaluated my husband, Dorinne saw his voiceprint and picked up on his high cholesterol. He had just been to the doctor who had told him that he had high cholesterol. I don't know how Dorinne does it, but there is something to that when you can evaluate a person's listening abilities and be able to pick out a medical condition or some traumatic event in a person's life.

Taylor has made so many changes. The teachers have noticed the difference and how tremendous it has been. He gets in the car and starts doing his homework. He can actually focus better and he stays on top of his schooling. It has just been a life changing thing. I'd like to say one last thing to Dorinne, "Thanks for giving me back my son."

STORY RESPONSE

Taylor's story is an important one because his issues encompass many of the advanced skill levels problems that are present in so many young and older adults today. He was only 13 when I first met him, but he was anxious, down on himself, and unsure of things. Yet a hint of "can you please help me?" showed through his façade. It is difficult growing up today if you are different. Kids can be cruel to someone who might think or act outside the box. I found Taylor to be a warm, caring, sensitive young man who enjoyed sharing about himself when asked, yet willing to help others with sincerity.

Although Taylor had been given the labels of OCD, ADHD, Tourette's syndrome, and dyslexia, all the labels didn't mean a thing to me when I sat down to evaluate him. I can only determine how I can help someone from my *DETP*. Parents often ask if they can send me copies of tests that have already been administered to try to limit their outlay of time and expense, but any other tests only provide me with extra information. They can not help me determine whether sound therapy can be helpful. My *DETP* reveals all the related pieces of *The Tree of Sound Enhancement Therapy* and provides clarity in understanding how sound therapies can be helpful. The title of the test, the *Diagnostic Evaluation for Therapy Protocol*, suggests that it is a test to determine a therapy protocol specifically for sound therapies.

Taylor's *DETP* indicated that 4 therapies would be supportive. It was suggested that he start with AIT, progress to Tomatis, move into BioAcoustics, and possibly revisit Fast ForWord if the need was still indicated. Prior to coming to me, Taylor had used the Fast ForWord program. This program helps speed up temporal sequencing skills which are important for the entire process of listening and reading. All too often, Fast ForWord is suggested without the understanding that there are other skills that need to be foundationally addressed first to achieve maximum results. This was the case in Taylor's situation. For him, Fast ForWord had been combined with the Wilson Reading Method. This can be very effective. However, Fast ForWord, as explained in *Sound Bodies through Sound Therapy* is at the *Leaves and Branches* level of *The Tree of Sound Enhancement Therapy*. One has to make sure that the *Roots*, *Trunk*, and *Body Maintenance* are well established and supported before going to this higher level. In Taylor's case, as with many similar cases, he learned and grew with specific skills from Fast ForWord. These skills became splinter skills or skill sets that can only be used to accomplish reading basics. For Taylor to fully integrate the sounds within words, words within sentences, and sentences within conversation, the foundational skills associated with the voice-ear-brain connection as set forth in my "Tree" analogy, had to be established first. In Taylor's case, this was accomplished by starting with AIT, then Tomatis, and followed by BioAcoustics. If Taylor continues to have reading issues, or if the need is demonstrated by my continued testing, Fast ForWord would then be suggested.

What happened with Taylor's tics was very exciting! BioAcoustics is the science of the future, of course, the future is now at *The Davis Center*. According to the creator of the BioAcoustics–Sharry Edwards, as of December 2004, *The Davis Center* is the only center in the United States offering BioAcoustics on a full time basis other than Ms. Edward's facility. Other centers incorporate the method into various practices such as massage therapy. *The Davis Center* offers BioAcoustics full time because it manages the *Body Maintenance* of *The Tree* analogy and stands on its own in order for us to accomplish the types of changes that occur.

BioAcoustics looks at the body as a mathematical matrix of predictable frequency relationships. Every body part and system has its own frequency or sound, therefore, we are combinations of sounds. These combinations are harmonious. When sounds are unbalanced, they become "out of tune" so to speak, and disharmony becomes apparent. Using a BioAcoustics vocal analysis we can identify the body's unbalanced frequencies and identify the baseline or core issues. In Taylor's case, his major frequency imbalance was related to Frequency Equivalent® of levadopa, something that ordinarily his body should be able to use to alleviate his tics. Once the Frequency Equivalent was introduced, Taylor's body was able to support his own natural form and function better, stopping the tics from occurring.

When Taylor stopped liking his sounds, it was time to return for another vocal analysis. The body is constantly changing and the voiceprint (when working on an issue) should be redone every 3 months. The repeat analysis demonstrated that Taylor needed to work further on issues related to his tics as well as supporting other issues. As with any sound therapy, it is important to understand that we can't wave a magic wand and make everything go away. The voice-ear-brain connection must be set in motion to allow self correction. The body needs time to adjust to change. Each adjustment is a part of the process that helps get to the core issue. Once Taylor dislikes his sounds again, it will be time to have them reprogrammed.

Some people wonder how someone with dyslexia could be helped with sound therapy. Again, only the *DETP* can determine who can be helped. In Taylor's situation, and in many others like him, the impediment is the inability to clearly hear finite differences between sounds. Some people don't understand that the inability to hear the difference between a /t/ sound and a /d/ sound can be quite significant. But for comprehension, this difference is monumental. For example, imagine hearing "You're bad, go to the closet", when in reality, "Your bat is in the closet" is what was said. Reading starts with the ability to hear differences between sounds. If the baseline isn't developed, the higher comprehension skills cannot be developed appropriately.

Taylor also was pleased with his changes from all of the therapies. His mother always said that there was "a special person" inside, and with our sound therapies this "special person" emerged. He is kinder to his family, gets along better with the kids at school, enjoys helping others, and feels good about himself. "I'm happier", he says. When his mother said, "Thanks for giving me back my son", she knew that sound therapy was special. Once again I saw how another "miracle" touched other lives.

CHAPTER THIRTEEN

Michael

ADHD
Central Auditory Processing Disorder

> "I saw monumental changes. I thought a parade should come to town to celebrate. I could hear and see the difference. His handwriting improved. His reading smoothed out. His vocabulary improved. His grades in school started to really improve. I couldn't believe it."

Montclair, NJ: Rose talks with a soft voice as she recounts the trials she and Michael had been through.

My son was born normal in every sense of the word. Pediatricians do a test for newborns. It rates their birth weight, height, breathing and color. They score them on all those things. It's sort of like a grading of normalcy. My son was fine.

Michael was a strong little boy too. You know how they prop babies up with blankets. They cocoon the baby in a blanket and prop them up so the babies can't move. Not Michael. The nurse said, "I move your son, and when I come back, he is on the same side as before turning him." The nurse thought she had forgotten to turn him until she caught him one day in the act of flipping himself. She just felt compelled to tell me that my son was going to be an athlete, "Sign him up for everything. I have never seen a three-day old baby do that."

When it came time to come home from the hospital, Michael fought me tooth and nail. You know how they buy those little outfits for newborns to come home in? Michael refused to wear it. He did not like having to put on that little sweater. He wore it once to bring him home. But I never made him put a sweater on again. He hates them to this day. He will not wear a sweater. I didn't know it then, but I subsequently found out that the sweater was irritating. It was too rough on his skin. This five day old baby almost beat me up so that he didn't have to wear that sweater home.

Michael had two ear infections in the first year of his life. We cleared those up rather quickly. Michael was born in April and he had his first ear infection in the fall. Then his second one came near his birthday. The first one, the pediatrician picked up on immediately. Being a new mom, I didn't even see the symptoms. Although I had switched pediatricians by the time the second infection came along, I took him to the doctor right away to be treated.

I did not intend to breastfeed my son forever, but he had his own ideas. We discovered he was lactose intolerant when I switched formulas. Michael started talking when he was 9-months old. The pediatrician couldn't believe how quickly Michael was talking in single syllable words. The mobiles that the pediatrician had hanging on his ceiling caught Michael's eye one day. Michael pointed at it and said, "birthday party" at age one.

At age three, I put him in a private school. When he came home the first week all excited about school, he was learning his alphabet. He got real excited about the letter "B." He was just so thrilled that he knew that letter and that he could write it. It was great to see him so excited. It was a Montessori school where each student got one-on-one time with the teacher every day for thirty minutes. This is why the kids really thrived academically, they just blossomed. It was a very stimulating environment and Michael loved it there. By October, Michael got another ear infection. The first two years of Michael's life, he had an ear infection every so often, but they were never drastic. This ear infection was different. It did something. All the excitement about school had gone away. He lost his focus and he couldn't tell you the letter "B" anymore. He lost it—it was gone.

I discussed it with the teacher, and she felt it was temporary. She thought he was happy at the school and he was getting along great with the other kids. He became a little social butterfly. I don't remember how many students were in the school, but Michael just loved having all those friends. My son is a real charmer. In fact, he wanted to go to school on weekends. He would get up and dress himself to try to go to school. It took awhile for me to get him to understand that school is only five days a week. The teacher thought that with all his new friends and the excitement of school, Michael would calm down and focus once he got over the initial enthusiasm.

Michael did well with numbers, shapes and colors, although he wasn't doing well with the alphabet. He stayed at that school for two years. They taught songs and he could sing the alphabet song, but he could not distinguish the different alphabet sounds. I didn't know that then. Neither did his teacher. The school was a very good school. They did a prescreening and Michael tested out at one hundred percent of what a child his age should know. However, Michael did not learn the alphabet the second year. The school was very successful at inspiring children to read. I have never seen a child who wanted to learn to read as badly as Michael did. But he just couldn't learn to read. So during the second year at that school, Michael's teacher came to me and suggested that I find a hospital that evaluated children. It just so happened that the hospital I worked at did just that. I made an appointment, but the appointment was six or seven months away. We had left that preschool by the time we did the evaluation because she also suggested that I put my son in a particular kindergarten. It would require us to move from one town to another. It was a public school which had an excellent reputation, however things change. I didn't get the top notch teachers for Michael and I didn't get the support that I needed. Michael didn't get the kind of support that his Montessori teacher thought he would. It just didn't work out well at all.

Michael had problems pronouncing things. He loved hamburgers, but he couldn't pronounce it. He would ask for a "hamver". At that time I didn't get it. Little kids say things like that all the time, and he got things confused. He called peanut butter, "mayonnaise". There were just so many peculiar things, but I just didn't understand what was happening with my son.

From age four to age five, Michael had three to four ear infections every year. He was on medications and off medications from October to April almost like clockwork each year. They were fast and furious. When we moved, we found a new pediatrician. To keep from missing work, I would be at the doctor's office at six in the morning. I would meet him opening the door. I would drop Michael off at the babysitter, go to work for a few hours, go to the pharmacy, pick up the medication, drop it off at the babysitter then go back to work. It was rough.

By age five, Michael had his last ear infection. The antibiotics cleared up the fluid and that was the end of that ear infection. They gave him a second round of antibiotics. Not because he had an ear infection, but because he had so much middle ear fluid. The antibiotics dried that up as well. I took him to an ENT doctor without a referral. He suggested not getting the tubes because Michael responded so well to the antibiotics. The tubes are a simple procedure and I think they should have been done, but the pediatrician agreed with the ENT. They didn't talk about it together. They just happened to agree.

Around the time Michael was almost six, we discovered that

he had hearing deficits. He had eighty percent hearing loss in his left ear and it was in that ear that he repeatedly got ear infections. He had them in the right ear too, but not as often. Instead of tubes, the pediatrician would only use medication on my son. I didn't know it at the time, but it was like Michael was hearing under water. When they gave him the second round of antibiotics, it cleared up the middle ear fluid, and he could hear much better. They evaluated him again and he was fine. He never had another ear infection again after that.

Michael hadn't been able to learn the alphabet previously, but now we were able to go through it in two weeks. Michael had been down about being unable to read, so I made it fun for him to learn. He was able to write his name. The kindergarten teacher had him put his name on paper, and he could write the words from memory. He had learned that from preschool. He seemed to draw it more than write it. When I realized this, I worked with him on it. Every night Michael would come home and we would go over the alphabet. When we got to the letter "Q", he thought it would be so difficult. He had been challenged so much that his confidence was very low. So I made the alphabet fun, and I made them animated. I asked him what he thought could be funny about the letter "Q". He said it was an "O" that was greedy, and was trying to eat the other letters, but it got a leg stuck in its mouth. That's how I taught him. I made it entertaining. We went through the whole alphabet in two weeks.

Michael's teacher wanted to hold him back a year and I agreed that he should stay in kindergarten. Michael was so set against it and I wanted him to get what he wanted. He had learned so many other things. It was only the alphabet and reading that were holding him back. So we worked hard on that. He succeeded and went on to the first grade.

Michael had a wonderful first grade teacher, but she didn't teach much of anything. He couldn't hear the difference between certain sounds, especially vowel sounds and some consonant sounds. He could distinguish the alphabet letters visually, but he couldn't reproduce the sounds of the letters when vowels and consonants were mixed together in word. He also couldn't distinguish between what he was saying and what other people were hearing him say. He couldn't reliably reproduce the sounds. He might say, "eat" one time and, "ate" another time. He didn't seem to know that what he said was wrong, or be able to distinguish what the other person said.

By the time Michael was in the second grade, he had learned to read a little, even though he still mispronounced words frequently. When Michael mispronounced a word, the teachers felt that he didn't know the word. They acted as if they had never seen anything like this before. They didn't help me understand this either. I told them everything that had been done. The teachers were horrible. They weren't trying to help him; it just got worse and worse. Michael would come home and cry. As a single parent, I devoted my evenings to coming home and doing homework with Michael. We didn't finish all the time, but we would work on his homework and that's how we spent was our nights together. Teachers just thought he was dumb or that was the impression my son was getting. They were doing rhymes and my son just couldn't get it. All my son's high expectations of school had been totally destroyed.

In the third grade, they did an evaluation. The only thing they told me from the evaluation was that he had trouble with vowel sounds. That was all they found. They started him in social studies. This was wild—the teachers determined that Michael's reading was two years behind, yet he did well with social studies. That just didn't make sense. He would come home with a report card that had all "F"s except in social studies and math. They classified him that year and put him in the resource room. Then they took social studies away! The first year, he had an excellent teacher. He did very well. Every day he got "A"s. But the problem with the resource room is that they teach very little. It was too easy. Michael had a different teacher year two and three. If he had had the same teacher for the other two years, it might have been different, but, it wasn't. He learned to read, but he still had the same problem with reliably reproducing the same sounds. He continued to have difficulties, although he was doing well in math.

Michael was placed in speech in the third grade. They did group sessions. One of the other parents told me about a great speech therapist named Phyllis. She took Michael on privately and she worked with him for two years. The child study team thought that I should leave everything up to them. They said they knew what to do with my child. I told them that I was taking him to a speech therapist and they laughed at me. The speech therapist wanted to talk to the child study team to find out what they were doing with Michael and how they were helping him. So the team took Michael out of speech since I had a speech therapist. Phyllis kept working with Michael. He improved. This shocked the child study team. They had told me that Michael would not improve. They thought it was an exercise in futility and that I would be sorry. Their philosophy was that people like Michael would still be able to graduate and make a good living, but they would never improve. How wrong they were. I knew how smart my boy was. I knew how advanced he had been. They just made me angry. At the end of the third grade, Phyllis diagnosed Michael with a central auditory processing disorder.

In fifth grade, they took Michael out of the resource room. Since the third grade I had hired tutors to help him with reading but he went through so many. They just weren't helping. I started demanding certain teachers in school, but the principal told me, "No." I had to go over their heads to the superintendent. That helped a little, but the teachers and the principal started resenting me. Every time the teachers got a chance, they would shift Michael out of their class. He was excelling, but the teachers said Michael was holding the class back and slowing them down. However, Michael was learning more. The teachers were really draining the energy from him and he would come home so stressed. He learned more, but at an incredible cost. It was a terrible price to pay.

He was to repeat the fifth grade in his public school, but I began searching for a different school. I had been looking for a private school and I found one in New York. My church had an affiliated church with a school in New York. Everybody was raving about the school and students were going from all over New Jersey. The school bused the kids there. So I looked into it. However, the school said they couldn't take Michael. Previously, the school had resources for kids with learning disabilities, but they had to cut them. In fact, the school is completely gone now even though it had been doing so well with the children.

However, before the school turned Michael down I was supposed to have had him evaluated at that school. I needed to take a few days off from work to take Michael to New York. The head nurse wouldn't let me have the days. A doctor at the hospital overheard me asking for the time off and asked me what was going on with my son. I described Michael's situation to her and she picked up on it right away. She told me about Auditory Integration Training and how it had helped other kids. I went home, researched it, and went back to work very excited about the possibilities.

So the summer before Michael repeated the fifth grade, I put him in AIT at a center in Connecticut. We finished AIT in August. Michael started fifth grade that fall. The school had scheduled him to be in support classes, but he didn't need support with reading, writing or spelling. He was able to leave all of his support classes within two weeks of starting school because he was doing so well. By December, however, Michael did a reversal and subsequently went into a depression. He sort of gave up for the rest of the year and waited to go into the sixth grade.

After his repeated fifth grade, I took Michael out of that school and put him in a small church supported school. It was the summer before the sixth grade and I started receiving materials about Fast ForWord, a therapy that helps with reading and easier comprehension of verbal information. Phyllis had moved away by this time, but she had put me on a mailing list that sends information to therapists. I am not a therapist, Phyllis just did it. I was receiving mailings trying to recruit me to learn Fast ForWord as a therapist. I started to look into it for Michael. I went on the Internet to find a therapist to do Fast ForWord for him. At that time, Dorinne was at *Hear You Are*. Michael was ten and he was in the upper age limit for Fast ForWord. After contacting Dorinne, I took Michael to meet her and do an initial evaluation for Fast ForWord.

The *Diagnostic Evaluation for Therapy Protocol* wasn't available at that time, but Dorinne picked up on some things about Michael that I didn't know. He could compare and tell what things were the same, but he couldn't tell what was different about them. Two fire trucks could have different wheels and all Michael could tell was that they were both fire trucks. He wasn't able to point out that the wheels were different. For that reason and a few others, Dorinne said that Michael would benefit from Fast ForWord. So we went ahead with it. Michael completed it and was able to do better at comparisons. I don't know that his reading abilities drastically improved. He was still two years behind as the experts at his school were telling me. But during the sixth grade, he made progress. He struggled, but he made progress. The classes were small so students had sufficient contact with teachers and Michael was able to improve a little.

He stayed there until the eighth grade. The public school had totally destroyed my child's confidence and I was trying to keep Michael in a private school as long as I could. Michael had tutors to support him in school. I reached out to Dorinne again in the fall of 2002. Michael was in the tenth grade. This time, she evaluated him using the *DETP*. She had advanced a great deal from when we first started years ago. Her "Tree" analogy was now in place. She found that Michael would benefit from AIT, Tomatis, Fast ForWord and BioAcoustics. I put Michael back in the public school and over Christmas break we started the ten days of AIT. I'm not sure if Michael had any improvement because he was out of school. Dorinne did a special session of AIT for us so that I was able to work and then take Michael to AIT after he got out of school. I didn't see much improvement. Dorinne explained that we were laying a foundation. We started Tomatis nine days later.

At the end of the first session of Tomatis, I saw monumental changes. I thought a parade should come to town to celebrate. I could hear and see the difference. His handwriting improved. His reading smoothed out. His vocabulary improved. His grades in school started to really improve. I couldn't believe it. What was the matter with people? Couldn't they see? He went right off the charts and kept on improving. We finished Tomatis in January. We did a second session in late March into April.

When they gave Michael his yearly standardized test, he scored across the board within his grade level for the first time in his history. He had a low score in language, but he was still in his grade level. He didn't pass geometry that year, but he passed it in summer school. Michael couldn't see the changes in himself. He was the last to see the changes that were happening to him. His math tutor was blown away. Michael was asking dynamic questions and he had never asked questions before!

Michael had been beaten up badly by the school system. His confidence was gone. So he was the last to see the changes taking place. He was doing phenomenally! Now as we were peeling away the layers of all of his disorders, we found that Michael had a real problem with Attention Deficit Disorder. It was clearly defining itself. Michael was very absent minded. He would leave things here and there. Dorinne suggested that Michael might have ADD, but now I was seeing signs of it. Michael finished the school year and I took him back to Dorinne for Interactive Metronome. It helped Michael harness his ADD. Michael did so very well with Interactive Metronome.

By the way, Michael is now an Eagle Scout, which we were proud to have invited Dorinne and her husband to the ceremony. I never held him back from anything. If he wanted to do something, I let him experience it. When Michael came back from Interactive Metronome, he returned to the Scouts. They took him skeet shooting and he did very well. That was another monumental change because Michael could now focus and gain his motor control.

Just this week, I was dropping Michael off at school. At the last minute, he turned to me and said, "Oh, I forgot. You have to sign this paper." I was thinking to myself, "What is it now? Is it some trip or something?" It wasn't anything like that. He had upgraded his writing class from a general class to an honors class. This was coming from a kid that two years ago had finally reached his grade level, having always been two years behind in the past.

Dorinne is a wonderful person. I am just so thankful she stuck with her goals. She changed our lives. Michael is looking at colleges. I knew it was there all along. I'm just happy Michael finally found it. I can't say enough good things about Dorinne.

Story Response

Reading Michael's story brought tears to my eyes. Prior to reading this story, his mother had not shared the part about his going into an Honors Class. Congratulations, Michael! Hard work on your part and well deserved.

Michael was one of my original clients at my old center, *Hear You Are, Inc.* He had received AIT initially from another practitioner. I first saw him for Fast ForWord. It was immediately apparent that Michael was a smart young man who was not able to demonstrate his intelligence. He had a wonderfully supportive mother who worked her hardest to get the best for her son. At the time when Michael first did Fast ForWord, my philosophy incorporating a sound therapy protocol was not in place, as I had not yet been trained in all of the therapies at the time.

I was very glad that Rose had Michael returned for the *Diagnostic Evaluation for Therapy Protocol* (*DETP*) even though he was in high school. He had received help with sound therapies in the past but the *DETP* could really help pinpoint the overall picture for him. He needed to repeat AIT because earlier results had not been retained. As I have indicated in *Sound Bodies through Sound Therapy,* and elsewhere in this book, it is by following *The Tree* analogy that maximum change can occur and be retained. Michael, having received AIT at an early age, did not know about the need to follow up with the other parts of *The Tree* because my protocol was not in place at the time. Fast ForWord was another sound therapy available to me at the time and it made sense then to administer it because of his test results and school functioning. Michael had needed something else in between AIT and Fast ForWord that was not apparent at that time.

The missing piece, when Michael first started therapy years

ago, had been Tomatis. *The Tree* analogy showed me that Michael had missed a big step between the *Root System* (AIT) and the *Leaves and Branches* (Fast ForWord) of *The Tree*. When warranted, the *Trunk* (Tomatis) is the crucial element that is needed for overall success. Michael had missed the *Trunk* segment when I first worked with him.

We needed to redo AIT because the *DETP* test data identified its need. I knew however, that he would not initially demonstrate very significant outward change. He was now laying the foundation for success by building on it according to *The Tree* analogy. I was not surprised that Rose did not notice significant change from the reintroduction of AIT.

It is the *Trunk* therapy of *The Tree* that lays the foundation for future growth and stability. Many of Michael's issues resolved once he was able to establish and develop the skills stimulated with this method. It not only helped him with reading, but it has also helped with his social skills, self-confidence, fine and gross motor skills. I have Michael on a videotaped interview saying, "I can now pick up a book and want to read to the end because I am able to understand what it's about from page one." Neither I nor the therapy taught Michael how to read. His body changed allowing his reading skills to develop. His ear was better able to hear and discriminate between speech sounds, process entire words with clarity and comprehension, and understand the subtleties of language nuances. When the body functions correctly, it can develop and learn skills more easily and appropriately, without distortions. Michael was finally able to take in and use all of the necessary pieces of what he was hearing, as well as what he was saying, to make sense of the world around him.

Michael's *DETP* indicated that a repeat of Fast ForWord

might be needed. I always phrase it that way, because sometimes the Tomatis method develops the skills that Fast ForWord may further refine. These skills are typically changed automatically with Tomatis and this happened in Michael's case. Once he was finished with Tomatis, Fast ForWord was no longer indicated by testing. Or perhaps it was that the skills that had been developed by Fast ForWord many years ago could now finally be put to use.

Interactive Metronome was suggested for a number of reasons. Even though attention was an issue, one reason Michael wanted to try Interactive Metronome was to enhance his athletic skills. Yes, Michael's attention had improved after Interactive Metronome. However, he also said he could throw a baseball better and shoot hoops better. For him, it had helped to accomplish what he wanted. For his mother, the therapies had succeeded in what she wanted.

The *DETP* also indicated a need for BioAcoustics. Michael was doing well enough after the other three therapies that BioAcoustics had been put on hold. Michael was maintaining the changes he made. Although as this therapy falls under the *Body Maintenance* section, it can be revisited at a later date if we find that he is not retaining the changes.

In the past, I had often encouraged Michael to consider college. The last time he was in my office, I was pleased and thrilled to be able to suggest an 8-day continuation program of Tomatis before he headed off to college. He now thinks more logically and is more focused in accomplishing all of his tasks. It was also an honor for my husband and me to attend his Eagle Scout Award Ceremony. All of us at *The Davis Center* are certain that he will continue to do well.

CHAPTER FOURTEEN

Eric
Autism, Sensory Integration Disorder
Central Auditory Processing Disorder

> "His articulation improved immensely. His skills in pragmatic language were greatly increasing. He was having better conversations and he was using words more resourcefully."

Northern NJ: Judy grabs cookies out of the oven and rushes back to the kitchen table. She sits down ready to share.

*M*y son was different from day one. He didn't want to be held, which made it difficult to nurse him. The only way I could console him at all was was to have him face away from me. I couldn't hold him like a normal child. He would scream constantly and he had an unbelievable amount of reflux. I had to change his sheets several times a day.

He had no play skills into his toddler years. You could bang a pot in front of his face and he would not react at all. It was as if a Martian had dropped him off at my doorstep. Eric was so totally different than any other child. He would drink out of the toilet and bang his head on the wall.

My son was diagnosed with moderate autism before the age of three. My primary intervention was a home-based Applied Behavior Analysis, which was both extensive and expensive. He had such a deficit in language, yet he could still keep up in school. That was mainly because of the Herculean effort at home. It's a huge undertaking when you have a high-IQ functioning individual that has such severe language processing issues. Because of everyone's efforts, my son has been mainstreamed since kindergarten. I used to have aides for him, but he no longer requires any. He receives no pull outs at all. He is your typical mainstreamed kid. He just has always had speech and language issues that make it hard for him to keep up in school.

Eric had multiple earaches throughout his childhood. A friend of mine whose husband had severe allergies was using a chiropractor. They suggested that I use their chiropractor for my son's earaches. I know it sounds crazy, but I decided to give it a try. The chiropractor helped a great deal. He helped my son's ears drain and he no longer had earaches.

My son was diagnosed at 9-years old with a moderate to severe central auditory processing disorder. At 11-years old, his diagnosis was upgraded to high-functioning autistic with sensory integration disorder. He had moderate receptive language delays and severe expressive language delays. Meaning, he can receive communications moderately well, but has a hard time expressing himself.

The point of all this is that my primary intervention with him was ABA. He would be considered a success story in ABA except for his speech and language, which was his main obstacle to successful socialization. His limitations in language were greatly straining his ability to assimilate or access teacher's instructions and his learning abilities as a whole. When you can't process information quickly, it limits your ability to learn. When you are constantly wondering what the teacher just said, you are missing out on basic understanding of what's going on.

Despite having spent hundreds and thousands of dollars for all of his therapies, I was very disappointed in the results I was seeing. Not only putting him through ABA, but speech twice a week, occupational therapy for an hour a week, Fast ForWord twice, over three hundred hours of Lindamood-Bell, the gluten-free diet and a full course of Tomatis with another provider. The cost of all these therapies was adding up and I wasn't seeing anything at all to make me proud or at least thankful. Although the ABA and Lindamood-Bell were useful in other ways, they did not help with his speech and language development. ABA brought him into being a functioning, happy child from a child who had been drinking out of the toilet and banging his head off the wall. If you look at the overall constellation of my child's issues, ABA was great. It just didn't help with my child's speech and language development.

The thing about my child that I could not tweak was his articulation, pragmatics, auditory closure and his auditory memory. What that means is that I could say three random, multisyllabic words and he could not repeat them back. When he was young, we had infinite hours of drill in front of the mirror practicing consonant sounds. That is a way to see how your mouth moves when you make certain sounds. That never worked. He couldn't remember even after such repetition.

I had seen Dorinne's advertisements for years and just never took them seriously until maybe two years ago. I went to a pediatric neurologist who recommended Tomatis, but she suggested another provider who was actually an Occupational Therapist. I tried her, but found limited success. My son found improvement in the area of sensory integration, but not in the area of speech and language. Recalling that *The Davis Center* provided Tomatis, I thought, why not?

So finally with nothing more to lose, I went to see Dorinne Davis. She evaluated my son when he was 11-years old. When Dorinne explained to me the *Diagnostic Evaluation for Therapy Protocol*, she suggested we do the Auditory Integration Training first. There were no earth shattering improvements, but I did see some changes in his maturity. I just didn't see any changes in his language development.

We followed AIT with Tomatis and then a booster. It was at this time that I saw great changes. My son's improvement was very novel. His articulation improved immensely. His skills in pragmatic language were greatly increasing. He was having better conversations and he was using words more resourcefully. The recent Tomatis sessions helped us get around the road blocks we had been facing with my son's speech and language development. Other than Tomatis, previously any improvements he had made had come with a great struggle. Nothing has ever been effortless for him—that was until the latest Tomatis session.

Other social skills were getting better as well. Eric was making eye contact and picking up social cues from peers. He is in the sixth grade now and much more discernment is needed than when you are in the first grade. Peers teach each other how to act and how to fit into their groups. My son was starting to understand the common group behavioral characteristics and he was following social rules quite well.

I wanted to know if there was a way to capitalize on the helpfulness of the microphone portion of the Tomatis therapy. The microphone portion had helped my son hear how he sounded by allowing him to hear himself talk. After considering my request, Dorinne found a way to do just that. My son now goes twice a week for an hour to basically do a modified Tomatis. His speech continues to improve, and the sophistication of his language is reaching higher levels. School is easier for him and he can keep up academically with little extra effort. He is also more successful socially than he ever has been.

The amount of assistance he needs at home is a quarter of what it was. Two years ago it was a strain for his teachers and classmates to understand what he was saying. He is not totally on target yet, but he is closing the gap. He is doing it effortlessly compared to how he struggled with it before. I have been able to make cuts in all of his therapies except for the modified Tomatis that he is doing now.

I wish I had brought my son to *The Davis Center* long before I actually did. I can see the improvements now and had I gone through it earlier, he could have been so much further ahead.

STORY RESPONSE

Eric showed great promise when I first met him. Initially, I met his mother Judy during one of our Open Houses, featuring our advanced *Read-Spell-Comprehend* program. She had explained her frustrations that night about having done so many therapies, including one of the therapies we offer, the Tomatis method. She was looking at *Read-Spell-Comprehend* to take Eric beyond his current skill level, and of course, to help him connect his academic skills with his speech and language skills.

As I typically do, I suggested doing a *Diagnostic Evaluation for Therapy Protocol (DETP)* to determine if there were any additional therapies that could support him in making further changes. Although he had done the Tomatis program previously, I still suggested the *DETP* because I sometimes find the need for intervention at other levels of my "Tree" analogy—levels that should have been addressed prior to the Tomatis method. This was the case with Eric.

Eric had issues with the one type of hearing hypersensitivity that is addressed by Dr. Bérard's Auditory Integration Training (AIT). It was important to retrain his acoustic reflex muscle to become more supportive for continued maximum hearing responses. This should be addressed by AIT, before attempting to address his listening problems. Listening problems are associated with the voice-ear-brain connection, which are addressed by the Tomatis method. AIT sets the stage for achieving lasting progress from the Tomatis method.

Judy had no earth shattering improvements to report from AIT. This is common for many people who need AIT. AIT helps develop better sensory input. Judy did, however, report changes in his maturity. What was really happening was that Eric was demonstrating a better understanding of what his body was taking in sensory wise, and as a result, he was better able to demonstrate that to others by his maturity. These changes had to be in place to allow the next step to occur.

The next step was to specifically focus on the body's response to all sound processing with an emphasis on the voice-ear-brain connection. Eric had problems with language because language messages were not being received appropriately at the brain. Further, there was a gap with expressive language and articulating speech. Once he started the Tomatis method at our center, heavy emphasis was placed on our "total person approach". I do not emphasize sensory integration or vestibular function by itself. I believe in integrating, evaluating and addressing all the pieces of the issues as presented in the entire voice-ear-brain connection. Judy began to notice the changes immediately. At first we emphasized the voice-ear piece for Eric, and then we added the brain portion of the programming to stabilize the results. Things finally began to fall into place now that Eric had the therapies in the correct foundational/developmental order. All of the pieces that all of his previous therapies had stimulated were now able to fall into place. It's like doing a crossword puzzle. You start working on the words you know, filling in as many words or letters as you can. You reach a point where you can't do anymore. You just need one letter to get the rest of the puzzle. In effect we supplied Eric with that one piece with AIT, and then helped him to fill in all the rest of the puzzle with Tomatis. The remaining pieces of the puzzle just fell into place.

Finally Eric can understand the pragmatic subtleties of language because he can better hear the rhythm, pitch, intonation, and intensity of the voice. He can pick up social cues better from peers because he is now better aware of body cues that were blocked out before. His peers' voices provide him with very important information that he was previously unable to discern.

Dr. Tomatis stressed the importance of the voice. It is the voice that is the body stabilizer. When moving through the Tomatis program, some people only need the basic program. However, many need repeated sessions emphasizing better voice usage and support. Such is the case with Eric. In Eric's case, I modified the typical plan to meet his specific speech and language needs.

The Tomatis method is a wonderful adjunct to speech therapy. By retraining the voice-ear-brain connection, as a listener and a speaker, a person feels more confident in what they are saying and how they are speaking. We have also helped other clients who were severe stutterers. Each person receiving the Tomatis method must go through the basic program. However, people with speech and language issues often need additional sessions to stabilize and enhance their voice-ear-brain connection in order for them to maintain its effects over time. People who stutter typically need additional sessions to reinforce positive speech production. What is important to understand is that the Tomatis method does not teach the person techniques to stop stuttering, to articulate sounds better, or to develop better language skills. The Tomatis method retrains how the ear and body process sound stimulation, which, after retraining, allows the changes to develop naturally from within the individual. The stutterer learns to adjust his own feedback loop. Articulation often improves on its own, and language evolves at its own pace. Do the individuals need supportive speech services? Often yes, to guide the progressing changes. However, some individuals need nothing extra. My staff speech pathologists work with our clients to support these changes.

We also offer guidance in the use of supportive home-based activities and therapies. For example, listening to Mozart and Gregorian Chants can be very supportive. Dr. Tomatis also developed "the listening posture", which is the key to success in supporting one's voice. I have heard of some people using a karaoke type machine as a way of supporting the Tomatis method. I strongly disagree with this concept because it does not support the internal listening concept that Dr. Tomatis encouraged. In fact, it emphasizes external listening and vibrational electronic sound, which for some, will reverse rather than enhance their progress.

The modifications we made to Eric's Tomatis programming emphasized the importance of learning to retrain the voice-ear-brain connection over time. Dr. Tomatis' third law emphasized that with training, the ear can be stabilized over time. We are very pleased with Eric's changes. As his mother indicated, the earlier brain change can be started, the earlier over all success can begin.

CHAPTER FIFTEEN

Kathryn

> "I am healthier, I am physically stronger, I am emotionally
> more stable, and I can express myself more clearly."

Great Meadows, New Jersey: Kathryn takes her time to recall things about herself that happened so long ago.

I felt that in the years I was growing up there was something amiss. I couldn't catch the beginning or ending of a word. I couldn't pinpoint if it was one or the other or both. I couldn't place what was wrong with me. I didn't know what it was and I didn't know how to go about finding out about it. I thought it just had something to do with a lack of intelligence or ability. Now I am a teacher. I deal with children with all kinds of problems, auditory processing issues and attention deficits. I know more about these things now.

When I was a little girl, I often had earaches. I remember having high fevers with temperatures as high as a hundred and three. My mother would be very worried and concerned. She knew something was wrong when she noticed that I wasn't playing. When there were no more noises in the living room, she would come into the room and see me curled up on the couch. I finally found out what the problem was. I had a hard ball of wax accumulated inside my right ear. I went to my pediatrician and he washed it out. I remember the ball of wax falling into the tin pan that he held under my ear. Then, I didn't have anymore ear problems. Now whether or not that had anything to do with my hearing deficiencies, I don't know for sure, but I think it might have.

My brother sailed through school with honors and then there was me with hearing deficiencies. When I was trying to take notes in school, it would upset me when I would try but couldn't accurately take notes. I had to rely on someone else to make sure I had everything I needed. It would embarrass me because I was a slow learner in many ways. I wasn't at the bottom of the group, but I wasn't at the top either. I was having trouble with reading, writing and listening. I was having difficulties with concentrating on material. My closest friends didn't seem to have the difficulties that I was having, although I didn't realize that I had these hearing deficiencies. Another thing that bothered me was that I had sensitive hearing. Background noises really were annoying. When I would be at a party, there might be music in the background and it distracted me. I couldn't concentrate on a conversation that I was having.

There was a part of my life that had to deal with my mother's problems. She had two nervous breakdowns and psychotic depression. It was traumatic for me to have to deal with that problem not knowing what it was exactly. It was never explained to me fully because no one wanted to worry me, but I was the one who had to deal with it the most. She would imagine things like what she saw or what people said. She was also on medications. My senior year of high school was my worst because her illness had escalated. I had little support because my older brother was no longer living at home. My dad worked all the time as a merchant in town. He had several businesses and had no time to be home. He was a good provider and he tried to deal with things as best he could. He always tried to get my mother help, which he did. When I was sixteen, my brother and I had a conference call with the doctor who had diagnosed her with schizophrenia, which was not the proper diagnosis. The most difficult thing for me growing up was her illness and trying to understand it. I did get some support from my grandmother and my aunt. I just didn't really talk to anyone else about it. My friends couldn't possibly relate. I didn't know what to believe because my mother would tell me things and I didn't know if they were true or not. I just felt lonely and depressed.

When I went to college, I learned I had some problems with comprehension as well. So they suggested that I take an extra reading course. I did, but I hated it. It was supposed to speed up my reading, but it didn't work for me. It did not help me at all. I wish that I had gone through *The Davis Center* years ago when I first learned that I had these issues.

When I was about twenty years old, I was diagnosed with an underactive thyroid. I had problems with maintaining my memory, my extremities would get cold and my immune system didn't work all that well. I always seemed to get colds and sinus infections easily. Of course considering I had been exposed to sick children since I began teaching in the public school, it was expected. I have gained some immunity to certain illnesses. Along the way I did get married, and the final blow from having an underactive thyroid was that I could never have children.

After years of dealing with all these issues, I was talking to a speech teacher at my school looking for answers to things that puzzled me at home. I didn't want to identify myself as the person in need of the information, so I fabricated an entire story about "a friend". I was a little hesitant to tell this speech teacher that the person I was describing was me, and that I was actually trying to learn about difficulties my husband seemed to have. He showed signs of auditory processing issues because I would have to repeat myself to him. I was basically asking a speech pathologist where "my friend" could go for help. She guided me to find *The Davis*

Center. I got on the Internet and went to their website. There was a lot of information that I read and studied. I saw all these therapies and what they did. I thought to myself, "This looks like some of the things I've been going through."

I contacted *The Davis Center* and decided to go forward with whatever it took. I had myself and my husband tested. I thought his test would be worse than mine, but mine was worse. Dorinne reviewed our *Diagnostic Evaluation for Therapy Protocol* with us and my husband decided that I should be the guinea pig. He said it was too expensive for both of us and he was skeptical about it in the first place. I decided to go through with it because I felt it would improve me in every way. I knew that it would help me on the job. Dorinne recommended I proceed with Auditory Integration Training first.

My goals were to desensitize my hearing and to possibly decrease the depression I was going through. My marriage was rocky, and I had been going through counseling, which turned out to be a waste of time. Had I known what I know now, we should have split up sooner. I was trying to combat depression with the therapies as well as work on my hypersensitivities to sound and allergies.

I started receiving treatment in July of 2003. I remember sitting in that little room listening to the specially filtered music. The first day, I felt a little nauseous and had a dull headache at the beginning of therapy. It didn't last long, and only lasted a few short days. Then after that, everything was okay. My sleep was definitely affected and the problems with sleep bothered me the most. I woke up early on most days. My sleep was definitely affected. Immediately after this two week session, I felt emotionally stronger but I still wasn't able to get a full night's sleep. My use of sound improved. My audiogram and acoustic reflexes improved. I was happier and more energized, as the therapies affect you entirely. Your brain, hearing and health are all connected. They had told me that sleep might initially be affected. Dorinne explained we were building a foundation. They told me that my sleep would return to normal and it did.

I went through Tomatis two weeks after AIT. Tomatis was different; it wasn't broken up like AIT. It was two or three hours at a clip. I had to listen to Mozart through the headsets. Dorinne decided that since I was going through some emotionally hard times with my divorce, she had me draw pictures of my childhood. I have pictures of different events that have occurred to me throughout my life. I have a picture of where I grew up in Virginia. I have a picture of my parent's house. There's a picture of a childhood friend buying me a soda. Dorinne told me that she wanted me to start with pictures of my childhood and then to bring them all the way up to the present. One of the more recent pictures was when I was in college and had rented an apartment. An even more recent one, was a picture of Lake George with my husband. We were sitting by a campfire and watching the boats in the lake. I am no artist, but it was good for me to focus on my childhood. I enjoyed this treatment and tried to make something positive out of it. Although with what I was going through with my husband, I had a hard time drawing that picture of my husband and myself. I drew pictures of the students in my class and one last picture was of a sunset, just a simple sunset. I also wrote a poem called "God's Boxes". It's just a little poem. "I have in my hands two boxes..." One box was golden for all of the good things in my life and the other box was black for all the things I needed to let go. I took stock of myself and thought about all the things I could list in the golden box and then all the things that needed to be listed in the black box. That was a good exercise for me because it helped me visualize all the things that I felt made me a good person and added fulfillment to my life. It also helped me to see what things I couldn't control and no longer needed to worry about.

After finishing Tomatis, I didn't see immediate results, but I did start sleeping better. It helped greatly with my depression as well as my memory. I am much happier now. When I used to go to bed, I would put my head on my pillow and I would hear these rushing sounds of air. That went away. I am not as sensitive to background noise. I prefer to be in a quieter setting rather than around loud noise, but background noise no longer distracts me from a conversation or from what I'm doing. I still have to cover my ears when the fire alarms go off at my school, although I am not sure anyone really enjoys the sound of a fire alarm.

Other positive changes that have taken place are that I know I am healthier, I am physically stronger, I am emotionally more stable, and I can express myself more clearly. I can express myself even quicker, rather than elaborate on long drawn out explanations. I think *The Davis Center* was an excellent support system for me. I got to know Dorinne. I felt like she was a friend more than just someone I was going to for therapy. The last time I went to *The Davis Center*, I had a test done. I hadn't lost any of my improvements. Dorinne told me that I had done well on the test. I am now dating someone with hearing issues and I am in the process of talking to him about going to *The Davis Center* for himself. I feel like I did the right thing even though I felt embarrassed at the beginning of this process. I mean, here I am a teacher and how could I have hearing deficiencies. At first I felt a little embarrassed and uncomfortable with talking about it. I've had to deal with these issues all my life and I feel good that I took the steps I needed. Even though it's like I'm starting over, you are never too old to improve yourself. Like I said, I wish I had learned about *The Davis Center* a long time ago. I would have done it all sooner.

Story Response

I always enjoy working with our adult clients. The feedback they give can tell you exactly what is happening. So often with our special needs clients, I have to rely on outsiders to report changes. The interaction with adults is always refreshing.

Kathryn and her husband at the time were an interesting couple to meet. They both were very curious about my philosophy and protocols, and of course skeptical of the entire process. As a former teacher, I am particular about describing the test results and how they relate to the individual in as easy to understand terms as possible. Because my approach is very different and I cover a lot of information, it can be difficult to absorb and understand all of the information presented.

As Kathryn said, she thought I would find more "wrong" with her husband than herself. It's not that I find anything "wrong" with people. My testing determines if I can make positive change for the person. Change for Kathryn just required more steps than for her husband. One reason I never guess about which therapy is appropriate anymore is that I am usually surprised when I see the results of my *DETP*. The integration of *The Tree* analogy is key to the success of my programs. When I began using sound therapy in 1992, I used the therapies only responding to the presenting diagnosis or symptoms. Now that my "Tree" analogy is developed, I have discovered it is a combination of therapies in the proper order that makes the most change and accomplishes my "total person approach". If the order is not chosen wisely, results take longer to accomplish and typically have reduced retention.

Kathryn's hesitancy to discuss her problems with her speech pathologist are not uncommon. Kathryn was in her fifty's when I met her. She had spent many years trying to understand herself and her relationships with others. She may have been depressed because of her inability to "take in" or to make sense of the world around her—this is an indication of a poor voice-ear-brain connection. This connection is essential to taking in sensory stimulation, emotions, and language. It impacted her relationships with her family, colleagues, and students, and it was a brave step for her to reach out for help. Thankfully her speech pathologist knew of our center and suggested that she seek out our information.

Kathryn's former husband never started therapy. Kathryn chose to start therapy and began to make change during a very difficult and tumultuous time in her life. She had hoped that the therapies would instigate the changes in herself that would alleviate some of the stress in her marriage. Of course, a marriage involves two people. The therapies helped Kathryn become a stronger individual. She now demonstrates the strength needed to make difficult decisions. The choices were always hers, but now she feels good about herself, is comfortable about her decisions, and is much happier. The process started with AIT by addressing the acoustic reflex muscle. This muscle supports the vibration of sound to the cochlea, but it also supports the vibration of sound to the vestibular portion of the ear. She experienced nausea because the therapy was stimulating this portion of the ear, our balance center.

One of the techniques that we use with adults who have had issues during development is to have them draw pictures of the events in their lives. Kathryn's pictures became an evolutionary collage of experiences in her life. The pictures she drew evoked an emotional catharsis relating to the various periods of her life. She was able to work through questions that she had about herself and foundationally build a stronger sense of self. I watched the "evolution of Kathryn". It was beautiful!

Kathryn has stopped therapy, but still continues to grow as a person. She is stronger and more confident about herself. I saw her for a one-year evaluation and was very pleased to see how well things have continued for her. I am very proud of her!

CHAPTER SIXTEEN

Kevin

> "He started improving eye contact and his speech was better. Overall, everything was changing for the better."

Absecon, New Jersey: Maria thinks back a few years to recall the facts about her story.

From birth, Kevin was pretty normal. He was looking at us and saying, "Momma" and "Dadda" at 15-months. A few months later, he was no longer looking at us and his speech went away. He also wouldn't respond to us. It was like he was going deaf. He started pacing when he learned how to walk. He would walk the floors back and forth; the kind of pacing that makes you nervous.

I put Kevin in an early intervention program, at a nearby hospital. We would go for two to three hours one time a week. They would have circle time and give kids a little snack. The people running this program were Speech Therapists, Occupational Therapists and Physical Therapists.

Kevin could only be in that program until he was three. His new pre-school handicapped program ran four half-day sessions per week. When he turned four he was placed in a full-day program. I kept him in the special school programs doing speech, occupational therapy and physical therapy. That was until there was a support group in our area that advertised a conference for kids with autism and various other problems. I was told there would be a lady at the conference that was doing the Auditory Integration Training right here in town, although she didn't do the testing the way Dorinne does. How can you do AIT like that? Where do you set the equipment? There are certain settings specific to each person. Without testing each person, how was it supposed to work? The thing was she was only a mile from my house, and it would have been so convenient.

I didn't know the lady didn't do individualized testing until I went to the conference. She had an exhibit table at the conference so I took the opportunity to introduce myself. I went up to talk to her and she didn't have time for me. I was looking for information from her. I couldn't believe that she wouldn't talk to me. So I said to myself that if she doesn't have time for me, then I don't have time for her and I walked away.

I did happen to meet another woman who had a child with all kinds of difficulties and one of them was a hearing sensitivity. She told me that the lady doing AIT doesn't do any testing and that I shouldn't go to anyone who doesn't test. I didn't know it at the time, but the lady I was speaking to was a speaker at the conference as well. She was an autism consultant and a nurse. I talked to her and she gave me a card because she did consulting on the side. I asked her if she could help me to see if Kevin was in a good program. She went to observe him at school and noticed a few things. Kevin stuck his fingers in his ears when a plane flew over the playground. He was also doing it in class when it was noisy. She observed that Kevin had a hearing sensitivity. She told me to see Dorinne, although I waited until the fall to take Kevin to *The Davis Center.*

Dorinne tested his hearing and did the *Diagnostic Evaluation for Therapy Protocol.* She told us we needed to start off with the AIT. While Kevin was going through AIT, I saw some behavior problems go away. It's hard to explain, but Kevin had shown all different kinds of behaviors, like pacing, fidgeting and not eating. He was different every day. These little behavioral problems started to go away. He was able to tolerate different foods that he didn't eat before. The different textures had always been annoying to him. Dorinne explained that it was all related. Tolerating different textures in his mouth are related to the ears and the bones in the jaw.

We went home after AIT and gave Kevin a break for two months. Then we began our first session of Tomatis. Kevin did well in that also. He didn't have to stay seated. He could walk around or do puzzles. He tolerated all the sessions well. He kept the headphones on his head, which was something that had been difficult for him during AIT. He wouldn't normally tolerate having things on his head. During Tomatis, he was very cooperative. His eye contact started to improve and his speech was better. Overall, everything was changing for the better.

We took a break for a month and then put Kevin through a second session of Tomatis. We had to do it within four to six weeks because Dorinne explained that it would work better that way for Kevin. Dorinne explained that if we waited eight weeks or longer, Kevin's hearing would relax because it was no longer being exercised, which would cause Kevin to regress. We went back for our second session of Tomatis and he continued to improve and he even seemed calmer.

Because of the success that Kevin had, we decided to put our other son through AIT as well since Patrick also had issues. He couldn't read in the first grade, and he had other things going on besides hearing issues. He was hyperactive and had a hard time sitting still. He was diagnosed with a communication handicap, which means he has issues with speaking, reading and paying attention. He developed fine with sitting up and walking. Everything like that was fine. He could function; he just was just having problems with communication.

If I would send Patrick to the next room to get something, he would forget what it was that I said. It was in his processing of information, and he'd only seem to hear part of what was said. For instance, he might only hear the beginning of what I said like, "Go downstairs…". He would go downstairs but forget the part about, "…and get the laundry basket". He would stand there wondering what it was that he needed to do or he would simply forget about it all together and begin doing something else.

When Dorinne recommended that we put Kevin through an 8-day boost in the summer, we also took Patrick and he did AIT. One of the major differences between Kevin and Patrick was that Patrick could tell me if he was feeling any different through the therapies. Kevin was eleven and he still couldn't talk. However Patrick was fourteen and he could tell me if something was wrong. When Patrick was younger, no one could understand him. I could understand him, but no one else could.

After AIT, Patrick could really recognize that sounds were painful and he started lowering the volume on the television and the stereo. He hadn't realized that sounds were hurting him. Now, he knew to try wearing ear plugs if the sounds around him were too loud. He also started doing his homework by himself. He started processing information better. Usually, I had to repeat myself several times for Patrick to understand. But after AIT, he could understand after the first time of being told. Overall he is more independent, more compliant, and is doing much better at school.

STORY RESPONSE

Upon meeting Kevin, it was apparent that his hearing sensitivities made him very anxious and nervous. The *Diagnostic Evaluation for Therapy Protocol (DETP)* test battery was instrumental in identifying Kevin's specific hearing sensitivities. This was important in addressing his overall ability to respond to sound. It was not surprising that his mother saw some of his negative behavioral responses disappear during and after AIT, because he was now able to receive better overall sensory input. He was now more comfortable with the world around him, simply because he understood its signals better.

As discussed in *Sound Bodies through Sound Therapy*, it is the indirect stimulation of the facial and trigeminal nerves through the ear that allowed Kevin to feel better about eating and to now try different textured foods. With better processing of his textural sensations, Kevin no longer felt certain food textures were painful or uncomfortable. It's like the gentleman who made the news recently because he had a nail in his head. He complained about headaches, but didn't know about the nail. His dentist's x-rays discovered a nail imbedded in his patient's head. Once it was removed, the headaches went away. For Kevin, once the excess sensory stimulation was diminished, he could enjoy different textures in his mouth.

Kevin's progress in Tomatis was very exciting. He began to connect much better with the world around him. As his mother reports, "everything was changing for the better". Kevin really began to blossom. He enjoyed being able to connect with others. He could now look a person directly in the eye and indicate that he understood what was said. With his new understanding he has also started trying to speak.

Patrick's changes were different. He was mature to begin with, yet he had subtle difficulties that impacted him in school and in everyday life. He began doing more things on his own and is able to read better. His overall comprehension has also improved.

CHAPTER SEVENTEEN

Final Response

> "Sound therapies make miracles happen everyday.
> From a child's first words to a stroke survivor walking,
> 'miracles' are possible."

*T*hank you for letting me share a few of the "miracles" that have happened at *The Davis Center*. They represent a very small portion of the many wonderful success stories we've had the distinct pleasure to be a part of. We have helped a range of cases from a head banging 2-year old autistic child become fully mainstreamed without an aide by the time he reached first grade; a thirty-three year old traumatic brain injured man have his first conversation with his mother; an extremely hypersensitive Williams syndrome child totally lose her hearing hypersensitivities; a Down syndrome child develop better communication skills; a severe stutterer stop stuttering; a stroke survivor gain better balance and motor skills, as well as improved speech and language skills; and so much more. We have also helped children enhance their giftedness and supported teenagers and adults achieve their true potential.

As you can see, people travel long distances to take advantage of our unique sound-based therapy approach. Our approach has been helpful to people who are severely autistic as well as for people who just want to improve themselves. Sound-based therapies have broad applicability.

People call and ask if I think that one of the methods would be helpful for their child or themselves. As you may have noticed, I work strictly from my *Diagnostic Evaluation for Therapy Protocol (DETP)*. It has become our signature approach to the use of sound therapies. It works! It is based on my concept of *The Tree of Sound Enhancement Therapy*, which is a developmental flow chart for the administration of all sound therapies. All sound-based therapies have a specific place on *The Tree* analogy.

Perhaps the only therapy I could separate from the importance of the total "Tree" approach is BioAcoustics because it stands on its own as a wellness therapy. I feel it is the science of the future. For *The Davis Center*, the future is now. With BioAcoustics, the use of sound is opposite to that of the Tomatis method, as it stimulates at the cellular level to make change.

The Davis Addendum to the Tomatis Effect developed from my research using my knowledge of the science of BioAcoustics and the Tomatis method, as well as my interest in spontaneous otoacoustic emissions. Everything about our development comes from the voice-ear-brain connection or the *Cycle of Sound*. Our inner self needs to be in balance with all external influences and stimuli. The voice reflects the body's stasis. If the voice is "off", then the body will reflect the discordance. Dr. Tomatis said that the voice produces what the ear hears and my *Davis Addendum to the Tomatis Effect* states that the ear emits the same stressed frequencies as the voice and by introducing stabilizing frequencies, the body can become better balanced. The body needs to be in harmony. If we think of our bodies as an orchestra, and our body parts as the musical instruments, when one instrument is out of tune, the whole orchestra is out of tune. We must stay in tune in order for all of the body parts to work in harmony.

Every Day A Miracle: Success Stories with Sound Therapy talks about many issues. I have included stories of people who have needed only one therapy and of those who needed many. I have also included stories of those people who had tried some of the therapies, before coming to me, with good or limited success, and I have tried to demonstrate through their stories, the importance of following the flow chart of *The Tree* analogy.

   The Davis Center will continue to compile many more compelling stories. I hope this book made you laugh, cry, think, and say "wow". So many changes are possible. Please share the possibilities with others.

Sincerely,

Dorinne S. Davis
The Davis Center
www.thedaviscenter.com

The Gift of Sound Fund

The Gift of Sound Fund provides scholarships for economically disadvantaged families and individuals in need of sound therapy. Through private donations, scholarship recipients are able to tap into the power of sound-based therapy for better learning, development and wellness for children and adults. Sound-based therapies include Bérard Auditory Integration Training (AIT), the Tomatis method (Tomatis®), BioAcoustics™, The Listening Program™ (TLP), Fast ForWord™ Series, Interactive Metronome® (IM), Samonas™ and more.

Sound is the Source

Sound is the Source is a non-profit organization dedicated to conducting valuable research and accumulating data on the benefits of sound's vibrational impact on the body. Innovative research methods will provide case studies for major medical conditions, including autism, AD/HD, APD, apraxia, dyslexia, hyperlexia, Down syndrome, Williams syndrome, learning disabilities, central auditory processing disorder (CAPD), health and wellness issues, and other minor learning/attention/focus related skills. The philosophy is that discovery and excellence in research will provide information for those in need.

For more information or how you can donate to *The Gift of Sound Fund* or *Sound is the Source* contact:

The Davis Center
1 Mannino Dr.
Rockaway, NJ 07866
Tel: 973.347.7662
Fax: 973.691.0611
Email: donations@thedaviscenter.com
www.thedaviscenter.com

Meet the Author

Dorinne S. Davis is the President and Founder of *The Davis Center*. An educational and rehabilitative audiologist with 35-plus years experience, Ms. Davis earned her Bachelor's degree in Speech & Hearing and Speech & Drama; then a Master's of Audiology/Deaf Education, both at Montclair State College, NJ. She is certified in Speech Correction, Pre-school Education, Speech & Drama, Teacher of the Hard of Hearing, and Supervision by the NJ Department of Education. She is licensed as an Audiologist in New Jersey, New York and Pennsylvania.

As an international lecturer in the field of hearing education and sound therapy, Ms. Davis has received outstanding awards and honors, which include recognition in over thirty *Who's Who* publications. She is also an active member of various professional organizations including, America Speech-Language-Hearing Association (ASHA), American Academy of Audiology, National Education Association, and the Educational Audiology Association.

Ms. Davis has various published works among them, the highly acclaimed *Otitis Media: Coping with the Effects in the Classroom, A Parent's Guide to Middle Ear Infections* and her most recent publication *Sound Bodies through Sound Therapy*, which set new precedents in the practice of sound therapies.

In the field of sound-based therapies, Ms. Davis is a certified practitioner in Bérard's Auditory Integration Training (AIT), the Tomatis® method, the Fast ForWord® Series and is a BioAcoustics™ Research Associate. She is a co-developer of Read-Spell-Comprehend®, and is trained in Samonas™, Interactive Metronome®, Earobics™, Lip-reading and Aural Rehabilitation, and is a certified provider for The Listening Program™.

Ms. Davis' research in spontaneous otoacoustic emissions and vocal analysis lead to the development of *The Davis Addendum™ to the Tomatis Effect*, further verifying a connection between the voice, the ear, and the brain as demonstrated 50 years earlier by Dr. Alfred Tomatis. Her work with sound-based therapies helped establish *The Davis Center* as the premier sound therapy center both internationally as well as in the USA.